THE FIELD GUIDE TO PREGNANCY

The Field Guide to

PREGNANCY

NAVIGATING NEW TERRITORY
WITH RESEARCH, RECIPES,
AND REMEDIES

CAYLIE SEE

LAc (FABORM)

North Atlantic Books
Berkeley, California

Published by
North Atlantic Books
Berkeley, California

Cover design by Bill Zindel
Book design by Claudia Smelser
Printed in the United States of America

The Field Guide to Pregnancy: Navigating New Territory with Research, Recipes, and Remedies is sponsored and published by the Society for the Study of Native Arts and Sciences (dba North Atlantic Books), an educational nonprofit based in Berkeley, California, that collaborates with partners to develop cross-cultural perspectives, nurture holistic views of art, science, the humanities, and healing, and seed personal and global transformation by publishing work on the relationship of body, spirit, and nature.

North Atlantic Books' publications are available through most bookstores. For further information, visit our website at www.northatlanticbooks.com or call 800-733-3000.

LIBRARY OF CONGRESS CATALOGING-IN-PUBLICATION DATA

Names: See, Caylie, 1976- author.
Title: The field guide to pregnancy : navigating new territory with research, recipes, and remedies / a book by Caylie See, M.S., L.Ac, FABORM.
Description: Berkeley, California : North Atlantic Books, 2016.
Identifiers: LCCN 2016009400| ISBN 978-1-62317-089-9 (paperback) | ISBN 978-1-62317-090-5 (eisbn)
Subjects: LCSH: Pregnancy. | Pregnant women—Health and hygiene. | Pregnancy—Nutritional aspects. | BISAC: HEALTH & FITNESS / Pregnancy & Childbirth. | HEALTH & FITNESS / Women's Health.
Classification: LCC RG525 .S414 2016 | DDC 618.2—dc23
LC record available at https://lccn.loc.gov/2016009400

1   2   3   4   5   6   7   8   9   SHERIDAN   21   20   19   18   17   16
Printed on recycled paper

To my loves, Adrian and Ava

....

Acknowledgments

I started on a path I couldn't have known existed in quite this way until one day I went down it and met all the people along it.

To my many patients, who were not just that, but were amazing, complex, and insightful individuals, it has been a privilege working alongside you toward your dreams of growing your families. You have influenced me greatly and given me the fulfillment and knowledge to contribute back in this way.

To my lovely partner, even though you had couvade during my pregnancy—maybe especially because you had couvade—your camaraderie, humor, and love hold me so deeply throughout any process.

To my daughter, who emerged during the writing of this book and unknowingly helped me with so many edits. You are the joy that everyone has talked about for all of these years. It is such an honor to be your mother.

To my dear friend and first editor, Joslyn Hamilton of Outside Eye Consulting, you guided me from gallivanting on a typewriter to writing an actual book. You organized my thoughts (and my cupboards). Going through this manuscript and our pregnancies together has been the most enriching editorial experience one could ask for.

To my team at North Atlantic Books, thank you for believing in this book and pursuing it with integrity, collaboration, and verve. It is a dream come true.

For everyone along the way, I thank you so much.

Contents

....

Preface

The Field Guide to Pregnancy is a personalized account of pregnancy based on my years of experience working with all types of moms-to-be (including myself). My two decades of practicing complementary medicine, along with my partnerships with Western medical doctors who specialize in gynecology and fertility, has exposed me to all sorts of stories and intimate details about many different kinds of pregnancies. Often, it is the challenges that stand out.

To get to the underbelly of some of the more common symptoms I hear about—as well as some of the more obscure ones—I've scoured medical databases that not all women have easy access to and combined the comprehensive information I've found with the experience I've gained working with thousands of pregnant women in my clinical practice. From this breadth of research and anecdotes, I've amalgamated information about the wide range of symptoms you can reasonably expect to encounter during pregnancy and what you can realistically do about them.

As a scholar and practitioner of Chinese medicine, I have always focused on women's health, with an emphasis on excavating the stuff that's not usually talked about and approaching solutions with moderation. Many of the recommended strategies of Traditional Chinese Medicine are taught from an ideal standpoint—not a realistic one. Because Chinese medicine treatments can be unachievable for the average Western woman, they are often simply frustrating and discouraging.

I believe things have to be doable to be effective. For instance, Chinese medicine often advocates strict dietary regimens, directing patients not to eat cold foods or prescribing exotic foods, instructions, which turn out to be nearly impossible for most of my patients to follow. Chinese medicine is ever evolving and adapting to work in a modern context, and I simply have not found it effective to force strict traditional regimens on my patients. Through my studies of Western and Eastern herbalism and nutrition, and simple observation of my clients and their well-being, I have learned that most ancient Chinese prescriptions need some balanced interpretation to adapt smoothly into our modern lives.

That said, the continuous thread from Chinese medicine that I *do* adhere to in my practice is the belief that women are inherently capable of taking care of themselves and their children in appropriate ways. In this book, I hope to empower pregnant women to let their instincts guide them and to balance their "gut feelings" with sound, integrative medical research in order to arrive at the very personal strategies and decisions one must make along the way while cultivating a healthy baby.

This book uses traditional strategies for a modern pregnancy, informed by the most useful research from Western medicine, to help pregnant women mingle intuition and time-tested remedies with information.

It is too simplistic to say that intention is enough to override very real symptoms, but staying connected to the original motivation to have your baby—while enduring discomfort and introducing or building on good habits in the face of discomfort and unknowns—can be a very powerful coping tool. Your pregnancy is an opportunity to cultivate your growing relationship to motherhood—all of the excitements alongside all of the intensities. This book aims to highlight your symptoms and things you can do at home to ease your unease. It gives you the tools to safely utilize nutrition, lifestyle changes, and helpful differential diagnosis for your self-care.

While I began this book from the clinical perspective of a medical professional working with moms-to-be, during the writing of this book I was fortunate enough to go through my own pregnancy, which made for a much richer account and some noticeable edits that I hope round out a professional and personal approach to pregnancy care. No purely academic experience prepares one to comment on the process of pregnancy; ideals can butt up against circumstance. Although each woman's pregnancy is completely unique, I'm glad to be able to incorporate invaluable direct experience to my advice and suggestions. In the pursuit of wanting to do everything we can to support our babies and ourselves, we can easily get overly idealistic and bypass simple pragmatism. Sometimes "good enough" is enough. Remember, part of health is happiness, and part of happiness is striving to do the best you can, while incorporating comfort and ease into your actual life.

....

Introduction

Every pregnancy is unique. Expecting women experience a wide range of symptoms, moods, physical issues, and perplexing questions during the ten-odd months of their pregnancy. Women's very personal experiences are up against a daunting societal and often arbitrary view of how they should feel during their pregnancy. Pregnant women consistently encounter not only glib, biased, and even inaccurate advice, but also frustrating, confusing, and disheartening anecdotes while they are either suffering their way through their pregnancies or genuinely coping and just looking to make well-informed decisions for themselves. This inherent conflict between what is happening and what friends, books, and even experts say can leave a woman absolutely distraught at the very time when she most needs to build trust in herself and her sources of reliable information.

We usually like to hold pregnancy as a celebration, and of course it is a wonderful life change, but it also potentially comes with a fair amount of grief and loss—the loss of who you knew yourself to be as a nonpregnant woman, the loss of your existing relationship to your body, and somewhat of a loss of control over what's happening *in* your body. This book aims to help you harness some of that control back by enabling you to make informed decisions and allowing you to indulge in the natural (but often downplayed) attributes of pregnancy challenges.

A redefinition of the self comes along with pregnancy; this book will help you outline and define your specific issues and needs. *The Field Guide to Pregnancy* normalizes the barrage of symptoms women experience without diminishing the importance or relevance of both the feelings and the symptoms themselves.

It can be terrifying dealing with the various symptoms and occasional maladies that go along with both healthy and high-risk pregnancies. Becoming a mother means that your new full-time job is to worry. But *The Field Guide to Pregnancy* helps you define what to worry about and act on in your pregnancy—versus what to learn to cope with. Pregnancy is a heightened time. It is often difficult to see the forest for the trees. *The Field Guide to Pregnancy* helps tease out what is a medically legitimate concern versus what might be subjectively concerning for personal reasons but not necessarily a cause for real alarm.

Medicine is always changing, and this book aims to equip you with the ability to evolve using smart decision-making processes. This is a handbook to guide you, comfort you, and support you from a place of compassion, pragmatism, research, and just plain, good advice.

Nutrition

From the time my own mother made my baby food from her garden, I have been a lifelong student of nutrition and the culinary arts. My own avid urban gardening and study of plant-based medicines have been fodder for the research and recipes in this book. I draw on the idea of dipping into your own kitchen, in order to find food-based approaches to supporting the different stages and phases of pregnancy and preparing you for all that pregnancy dishes up, as well as a healthy birth, recovery, and life.

Nutrition is of the essence, and "you are what you eat" is never as true as it is when you have a developing baby inside you. The foods you choose will nourish and help determine not only a healthy pregnancy but also your child's long-term health. The raw materials you consume become nourishment for you and your baby. Eating high-quality foods helps both of you derive the best potential from your health, and this book will give you choices to make and use as a basis for your own creativity and tastes.

Each recipe in this book assumes these general principles for you to follow when concocting your pregnancy foods:

- Choose organic foods whenever possible.

- Minimize the pesticide, chemical, or hormone exposure (such as from nonorganic meats) to give your body the best opportunity to send resources to baby.

- Lean toward eating more locally and seasonally—principles in alignment with Chinese medicine's penchant for attunement to your environment as a state of optimal health.

Any good, replicable recipe is usually based on a little bit of science and a little bit of intuition. Pregnancy is no different. Although there's no tried and true recipe for everyone, there are ingredients that people can modify to their own tastes to incorporate into their nourishment. I'll talk about nutritious ingredients for each stage of pregnancy and offer up recipes throughout this book for you to modify as you see fit.

Supplementation

The use of plants as medicine is as old as mankind, which means it's as old as the act of giving birth. Supportive eating can be as important or even more profound than taking supplements or even medications. However, there is certainly a time and place for supplementation, and *The Field Guide to Pregnancy* helps guide you through safe and thoroughly considered approaches on the gradient from lowest to highest interventions.

Western and Chinese Stages of Fetal Development

Often, pregnancy manuals include clinical illustrations or photographs of the developing embryo and fetus. I've opted against this type of visual size comparison in this book. You'll know your baby is growing because your stomach is growing—and you may be having ultrasounds as well. I think it is more useful to picture your baby *as a baby* and begin to connect with the growth inside you in that way. Having a baby can be abstract and daunting enough without comparing it to a "grape" or a "raspberry" or any other fruit.

Personally, I don't think it's helpful imagining birthing a pineapple. So, I'll give you the normal growth ranges, which you can compare at your prenatal visits. You can also utilize the at-home measuring technique (see sidebar on page 55) to interact more with conceptualizing your baby's size as it grows. Each chapter also begins with a helpful infographic for a glimpse of the latest pertinent developments with baby.

Chinese medicine is founded on the idea that the principles of nature are reflected in the body's physiology, with very specific correlations between elements in nature and fetal development, which explain certain symptoms and tendencies during specific phases of pregnancy. In alignment with the idea of looking to nature for information and resolution of discomfort, Chinese medicine encourages you to draw on natural (plant and food-based) remedies to tend to pregnancy symptoms.

From a Chinese medicine point of view, imbalances fundamentally occur when we are not in harmony with nature. In the context of pregnancy, that really means being attentive to your *own* nature and learning to identify your unique personal needs and incorporating healthful ways to attend to them.

Each chapter of this book commences with a detailed description of the relationships of the Chinese organ systems to the stages of fetal development. Familiarity with this Chinese pathophysiology affords an understanding of the ways symptoms that we know about in Western medicine occur from a Chinese medicine perspective. The two models together can help us see why certain symptoms arise and correlate the symptoms with diet and lifestyle advice to address them and provide some insightful guidance on further caring for you and your baby during each month of pregnancy.

I find the Chinese medicine model helpful for bringing in a more comprehensive view of your pregnancy stages and using some of the figurative associations as a launching pad for understanding what's going on in your body and how to care for yourself. So as not to be too confusing, throughout the book, I capitalize the Chinese organ systems and lowercase the Western systems:

CHINESE MEDICINE	WESTERN MEDICINE
Liver, Heart, Spleen, Lungs, Kidneys, etc.	liver, heart, spleen, lungs, kidneys, etc.

General Recommendations

Being a practitioner of Chinese medicine is also about recognizing someone for who they are and what is right for them as an individual. This is
why I don't just recommend blanket acupuncture treatment protocols and
herbs for everything and everyone! Being a Chinese medicine practitioner
has exposed me to many methods of healing and treatment, and I draw on
all of these modalities to give you options to pull from and experiment with
to see what's a good fit for *you*.

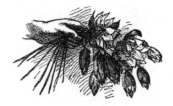

Month One
Changing

A Preface to the Weekly Developments

For a brief revisiting of the birds and the bees, the start of your menstruation begins week one of your cycle. In week two, fertilization occurs and in week three, the fertilized egg (blastocyst) implants in your uterus, and the amniotic sac begins to form. So, when you take a pregnancy test (about two weeks after ovulation) this is actually considered week four of pregnancy (see the sidebar "Did You Know: You're actually two weeks further along in your pregnancy than you may have thought?" for more information).

And of course for all of the upcoming weeks of your pregnancy, it is important to bear in mind that developmental markers are approximations. There's a broad spectrum of what constitutes normal, and every baby develops at his or her own pace, to some extent. So, take these as guidelines to help you continue to investigate your pregnancy.

WEEK FOUR

- Neural tube is formed.

WEEK FIVE

- Embryo is .13 inches.
- Brain and spinal cord begin to develop.

- Major organs begin to form as well as the digestive, nervous, and circulatory systems.

....

WEEK SIX

- Baby is about .25 inches.
- The heart and major blood vessels are developing, and the beating heart can usually be detected during an ultrasound.
- The face, hands, and feet start to develop.

....

WEEK SEVEN

- Baby is .51 inches.
- Over 100 brain cells are produced each minute.
- The heart is becoming more complex.
- The kidneys are forming.
- The arms and legs begin to appear, and joints start to develop.

....

WEEK EIGHT

- This week, baby is officially called a *fetus*, which means "little one" in Latin.
- Baby is .63 inches (and growing a millimeter a day) and has a measureable weight now of .04 ounces.
- In case you didn't know that there was one, the tail is now gone.
- Taste buds are developing.

....

East-West Fetal Development

The first eight weeks of gestation are correlated with the Chinese Liver. Associations of the Liver system include the element of wood, the color green, the eyes, and bitter flavors. The Liver's nature is the springing forth of new life (think trees and plants bursting in the springtime).

Did You Know: You're actually two weeks further along in your pregnancy than you may have thought?

It can be confusing to find out you are "four weeks pregnant" when you're pretty sure you only conceived about two weeks ago. Four weeks ago, you were probably even having your period.

For a little insight, let's harken back to the idea of Chinese medicine's observation of nature as it's applied to the body. Before there were ultrasounds, women looked to the lunar cycles to understand when they would give birth. After they suspected they were pregnant, women would note the phase of the moon that they saw in the sky and expect to give birth after seeing that same phase ten times. Ten lunar months is about 295 days, whereas Naegele's Rule (Naegele was an obstetrician in the 1800s who developed the modern standard for calculating due dates) states that an average pregnancy lasts 280 days (forty weeks).

To compensate between the lunar calendar and Naegele's rule, we count from the first day of your last menstrual period, which adds about fifteen days—the approximate time between menstruation and ovulation—to the total time of pregnancy. So by the time you miss your period and suspect you might be pregnant, you're already about four weeks along!

Obviously, this is an imperfect system, since menstruation and ovulation dates vary from woman to woman, and implantation doesn't even occur until seven to ten days after ovulation (and even sooner if you've gone through IVF because some of the cellular division has already happened by the time you transfer the embryo), but this should explain why you're being told you're four weeks pregnant, and why your due date will probably shift throughout your pregnancy as different measurements and assessments are taken. Interestingly, if left to their own devices, many first-time moms will go about two weeks past their "due date"—which brings us back to the original lunar cycle.

Drawing on the associations and the nature of the Liver, one supportive technique for this stage is to take walks in beautiful places and soak in nature's calming attributes. Not only is this a good way to get some endorphins going and destress, but being around fecundity is particularly nourishing during this Liver-driven time. Additionally, looking at beautiful greenery at this green stage in your own pregnancy is a great way to reflect on the recent changes to your body and life and to begin to move through them gracefully. The Liver system also goes right into the reproductive tissue. So, activating the Liver through activity promotes blood circulation, which brings nourishment to your baby.

We can also think of this Chinese Liver as being loosely related to our Western nervous system. In fact, in fetal development (from both an Eastern and Western perspective), the nervous system is exactly what's forming during this time: baby's brain and spinal cord are already beginning to develop.

Just as you and baby are merged together, in Chinese medicine, emotions and physiology are intimately paired. The first month, while baby's nervous system is beginning to form, is a great opportunity to work on your own nervous system. Tending to your own potential stress during this new transition supports you as well as baby. You can also think of this time as an opportunity to develop connections to yourself, to your baby, and to your new life.

These first weeks are the beginning of many changes to come. So, building up some supportive tools can help you set the precedent for navigating your pregnancy. It's a wonderful time to focus on self-nurturing and self-care and to set the rhythm for the journey ahead of you.

Confirming Your Pregnancy

Most women suspect pregnancy around a missed period and confirm with an over-the-counter pregnancy test. The first such test was introduced in 1976, and although the technology to sensitize the test has improved, the results can occasionally still be false-negative or even, very occasionally, false-positive (if this happens you need to look at other hormone-related issues with your practitioner). It is more likely than not that if you've taken the test fourteen days or more after ovulation, your test is accurate—no matter how many times you stare at it. If you'd like a more quantitative test (just how pregnant *are* you, anyway?), you can request a lab test from your physician to look at the amount of human chorionic gonadotropin (hCG), better known as "the pregnancy hormone," in your blood.

If you have a blood test for initial hCG levels, it's comforting for the number to be larger rather than smaller (let's say between 1,000 to 2,000 mIU/mL), but bear in mind that it's more relevant that this number doubles or at least significantly increases from the initial blood draw to the next one. (A second blood draw is sometimes taken two days after the first one if there's a question about the initial number or to confirm an appropriate increase.) The variance in the numbers (sometimes initially quite low) and the growth of the number is great, but not solely enough of a predictor for success. So, if it's looking a little wobbly, hang in there. It's too soon to know what's going to happen. The best you can do is delve into supporting your pregnancy.

And if you are scrutinizing symptoms looking for confirmatory signs, know that it usually takes a few weeks for significant pregnancy symptoms to set in. Just stay with what you know right now. You've had your first positive pregnancy marker, and you're pregnant right now. I would also like to emphasize that there's virtually nothing you can do to disrupt a viable pregnancy. So, do your best to hang out with the unknown and tend to yourself as well as you can.

The Shock of the New

At a time when you may be feeling a bit of shock and craving some familiar comforts, your usual creature comforts may be on the "banned" list—things like coffee, wine, and hot baths are all but forbidden during pregnancy. It's time to look for some new indulgences that will help you find some ease, nurturing, and nourishment when you need it most. It's not just about baby; it's also about tending to you. I highly recommend quiet yet busy activities such as walking, or just being in nature, gentle yoga, meditation or guided imagery, reading, cooking, knitting, or other crafty work—and an occasional cup of hot cocoa—to help you unwind and cope with the stress. These activities can help you feel like you're doing something good for your pregnancy even if you're feeling a little lost.

Indeed, emotional shock can often be the very first symptom of pregnancy. Change, after all, is often disconcerting—especially such an incredible change as finding out that you're pregnant. Even if you've been planning this pregnancy, it can be truly traumatic to find out you're actually pregnant. It's probably the biggest news you'll ever get in your life, and it affects your whole life indeed. So, be gentle with yourself as you adjust to this huge change. It is okay to not fully connect with your pregnancy right away. That's normal. It's like any other relationship: it takes time to acclimate, build trust, and understand this new dynamic in your life. You have plenty of time to grow into the idea (literally).

For women who have had a hard time conceiving, the nervous system can be patterned around peaks of hope and dips of grief during each previous cycle. It may take some time to reestablish a trust in your body and to adjust and connect with the new paradigm of pregnancy. I like to think of this as "repatterning." In a therapeutic paradigm, one approach to trauma or a place of stuckness is to consciously and incrementally intervene. Similarly, in this stage of your pregnancy, you are seeking to create new and healthy thought patterns. Now that you're pregnant, it's an opportunity to reevaluate what your pregnancy journey means for you and to start to connect, even in the face of risk, with the new life developing in you. It's time to let go and let nature get to work, and it's okay to feel nervous. You are not harming your pregnancy by feeling any and all of your feelings.

But as we are thrust into this state of intense flux, it can be very confusing to try to simultaneously indulge in the joy of being pregnant while battling so many uncomfortable symptoms. You might not even feel pregnant. You might feel simply *sick*. Since nothing in this process is black or white, this, as with the rest of your mothering, will be about continually building a relationship with discomfort and listening to and trusting your intuition. So, give yourself room for "normal nervous."

Aside from morning sickness, many physical surprises may happen in the beginning stages of pregnancy. Already, your digestion is slowing down to accommodate your pregnancy, and your body's hormones are making massive adjustments. It's not unlikely that you will experience insomnia, fatigue, or even lethargy; sore breasts; bloating. There are also more intense symptoms that can arise such as vaginal bleeding, abdominal pain or pelvic pain and odder symptoms such as a metallic taste in your mouth. I can't tell you how many times women have come into my clinic saying, "No one told me I would feel this (fill in the blank) way!" Seemingly overnight, competent, energetic, productive women are often converted to forgetful, exhausted couch potatoes.

If this sounds familiar, you are not alone! I can assure you that it's no reflection on your abilities as a mother or a woman, nor does it necessarily speak to your level of self-care. This is just nature taking over. Your body is doing the tremendous work of building a baby, and it's time for you to slow down. Since most of us have a hard time modifying our lives voluntarily, nature has a nifty way of making us do what we can't or won't do for ourselves.

Nutrition

Now that the seed has been planted, so to speak, it's a great time for the seeds for healthy eating to be tilled as well. We've all heard the expression "eating for two," but although you will probably find yourself eating more than usual, you won't necessarily be eating double the amount that you're used to. You should, however, at least double your nutrients and your level of self-care. I think of it like companion planting—a gardening technique that strategizes which plants can be planted in proximity to each other to optimize nutrients and contribute to growth. Like in a companion garden, you and your baby are two people coming together and beginning a symbiotic relationship of shared nutrients to promote the best yield for everyone involved.

As soon as you know you are pregnant, it's important to start eating in a way that is nutritious *and* doable for you. Of course, this can be challenging when coupled with morning sickness (more on that later). Recipes with (I hope) palatable morsels are sprinkled throughout this book to support you and your baby throughout the pregnancy. As we move into what to eat, let's start with what *not* to eat and build from there.

Foods to Avoid to Prevent Foodborne Illness

For the most part, pregnancy is a great time to follow your instincts about food and eat what you feel like eating. But there are certain foods that pregnant women should avoid. It's important to minimize exposure to foodborne microorganisms at this time, because your immune system is slightly suppressed during pregnancy—partly to reduce the chances of your immune system rejecting your growing baby.

Aside from personal aversions and what you might already feel inclined to reject, here's a list of the main cautionary items you should avoid. However, If you do get a food-induced sickness, be comforted by the fact that food poisoning rarely affects the baby's health.

- High-mercury seafood and shellfish: You can check with your local fish advisories to stay current, but this typically includes albacore, halibut, trout, tuna, salmon, and oysters, as a starting place.

- Raw or undercooked eggs, which are also found in eggnog, batter, hollandaise sauce, and Caesar salad dressing.

- Raw fish and raw meat

- Refrigerated pâtés

- Unpasteurized cheese (brie, feta, Camembert, bleu, ricotta, queso blanco, queso fresco): Pasteurization kills *Listeria monocytogenes,* which is a likely agent in bacterial infections during pregnancy (see Listeriosis on page 83 for more information).

- Juiced Brussels sprouts: Contain isothiocyanates that can induce chromosomal changes in cells and potentially cause damage to a developing baby.

- Alcohol

- Preferably eliminate, but at least minimize, caffeine, including not only coffee, but also mate and some herbal teas (black tea, green tea, guarana, kola nut, betel, bitter orange, yohimbe, mangosteen).

Herbal Tea

During a time when coffee, black tea, green tea, alcohol, soda, and even too much juice are not optimal, what's left? Herbal tea can be a comforting treat for women, but—alas—not every herbal tea is safe. Even some of the typical remedies we see on the market for pregnancy have controversial ingredients. The lists below can help delineate what to absolutely avoid versus what to drink moderately, and what you can drink regularly without any concern.

Herbal teas that should be avoided in straight form during pregnancy are:

Aloe	Anise
Black cohosh	Black walnut
Blue cohosh	Fennel
Lime blossoms	Catnip
Comfrey	Dong quai

Ephedra	Ginseng
Hibiscus	Horehound
Kava root	Lemongrass
Licorice root	Mate (often contains as much caffeine as
Mistletoe	coffee)
Mugwort	Pao d'arco
Pennyroyal	Rosemary
Sage	Sassafras
Saw palmetto	Senna
Vetiver	Wild yam
Wormwood	Yarrow

In addition to the above "avoid" list, there are a few herbs that are a mixed bag, but bear in mind, the dose of herbs in a normal cup of tea is unlikely to have any negative impacts. This is just for you to be equipped with the full picture to choose to be as conservative or lenient as you'd like:

- Chamomile: Some people who have plant or seasonal allergies can also be allergic to chamomile.

- Ginger: Ginger's function of easing morning sickness, which, by the way, takes about three weeks to kick in, has been substantiated in multiple studies as a safe and effective option, but there's also some conflicting evidence that early on in pregnancy it may negatively affect fetal sex hormones.

- Nettle: This is a great iron builder and is likely very safe after the first trimester.

- Raspberry leaf: Likely safe after the first trimester, but has shown conflicting results in terms of both preventing, but also potentially stimulating, uterine contractions.

- Rose hips: A great source of vitamin C and can be safely consumed after the first trimester.

....

DAILY PREGNANCY TEA

It's tea time, and you may be thinking so, what *can* I drink? It can be confounding to try to take care of yourself *and* stay hydrated *and* simultaneously avoid so many beverages.

Here's a safe pregnancy tea for daily consumption:

Mix equal parts cinnamon, lemon rinds, and lemon balm steeped in a cup of hot water with some honey.

....

TAKING ROOT SOUP

I always turn to this soup as a first step in nourishing a new pregnancy. It's a great way to get in the swing of making bone broth, which can be a wonderful companion during and after birth, and I love the idea of rooting with roots. It's as easy as one, two, three ... four.

Ingredients

1 pound organic, grass-fed beef, cubed

2 turnips, ½" cubes

3 parsnips, quartered

4 carrots, ½" slices

1–2 tablespoons Sesame oil

Sea salt

Bone stock 3 cups (see Boosted-Up Chicken Stock recipe, on page 46)

Directions

Coat the beef cubes in a generous covering of sesame oil and season with sea salt to taste.

Place pot (or Dutch oven) on stovetop and set flame or temperature to medium-high, add beef and sear all sides until brown (approximately five minutes). Add vegetables and stir periodically until starting to soften. Pour bone stock into pot and cover. Either turn stove down to a simmer for forty minutes, or place Dutch oven in the oven and cook at 250 degrees for two to three hours.

....

Insomnia

You've woken up to find that you're pregnant, and now it may seem like you'll never sleep again! Most people can't fathom how they will survive these initial disrupted sleep patterns, let alone the sleep changes that will occur once the baby arrives. The "good" news is that nature has a way of making you practice sleep deprivation long before the baby comes. The even better news is that you *will* get through it.

I like to call this phenomenon of early-pregnancy insomnia "nature's preparation." Pregnancy is a time to begin to acclimate to the impending changes in your life once you have a child. Sleep disruption is most typical in the first trimester and the third trimester—and, of course, postpartum—but evolution has craftily made babies quite cute, and made you innately bonded to them, so that when they inevitably wake you up at night, the lack of sleep fades into the background, and you do what needs to be done to love and nurture your little one.

In the meantime, it can be daunting to feel sleep deprived long before your baby is even here to keep you up at night. Although there is no known explanation as to why nature is full of such ironies, we do know that sleep disturbances occur as a result of physiologic, hormonal, and physical changes associated with pregnancy. For instance, the need to consistently get up and urinate certainly can affect sleep. If you already have an existing sleep disorder, pregnancy may also exacerbate that pattern.

Let's face it. Anyone is bound to be strung out without enough sleep. However, severe sleep disruption may warrant going to a specialist for appropriate diagnosis and treatment. Having this evaluation prior to birth may help minimize the potential for postpartum depression as well. It's a good idea to assess the impact your lack of sleep is having on your life and take it from there.

But to palliate your initial sleep changes during this formative period of pregnancy, you may want to try a guided audio relaxation to help lull you back to sleep in the wee hours. By the way, this is a great time to record any active dreams you may be having. Many women enjoy looking back on their vivid pregnancy dreams as their own private storyline of their pregnancy. These dreams can often be a portal into examining some of your subconscious fears, anxieties, and hopes about your pregnancy, mothering, and intimate relationships.

Depression and Anxiety

Depression and anxiety, which I consider spectrums of each other, are complex issues, and the gradient of severity can be great. My general advice is that whatever tips the scales in one direction or another for you is worth seeking support around, but if depression and anxiety are arising for the first time during your pregnancy, do take into account that it is normal to have large feelings surrounding this big event.

Attempt to not compound the existing feelings by adding worry into the mix. Instead, try to give yourself permission to feel the full extent of what you're feeling and move slowly, with an emphasis on observing rather than changing your state. Combine this emotional stillness with physical movement such as walking, and if this initial approach doesn't settle you a bit, seek out whatever levels of support feel right—more time with your partner, regular meet-ups with friends or family, massage, acupuncture, talk therapy, or even psychiatry to explore the potential of help from medications.

Fluid Changes: Bloating, Swollen Breasts, and Increased Urination

Fluid changes abound right now, so it's a deceptive time in that you might feel like the retention—or "fatness"—already calls for maternity clothes. What's actually happening is that progesterone from the placenta is in full swing, and this same hormone that's favorable for implantation also mimics symptoms of premenstrual syndrome (PMS) such as bloating and breast tenderness.

Progesterone also relaxes smooth muscle tissue in your body, including in your gastrointestinal tract. This relaxation isn't so relaxing for you since it slows down digestion and metabolism, which is another contributor to bloating and flatulence. Not to worry—after the first month of distention and discomfort, your bloating will probably start to recede, and you'll enter a pregnancy weight that actually represents the baby's growth. As for the other discomforts, sluggish digestion does continue to increase throughout

Did You Know That There Are Nonpharmaceutical Ways to Combat Insomnia?

The only thing you can control (usually) is your breathing. So, focusing on your breath can be a great way to connect with safety when you're feeling out of control. Meditation and Mindfulness have been shown to help with both falling asleep and waking up.

A basic technique is to focus on the rise and fall of your breath: inhaling and expanding your lower belly, then exhaling and gently pulling your lower belly toward your spine. Every time your mind wanders (which may be every millisecond), simply return to focusing on the rise and fall of the inhale and the exhale. Try a cycle of ten minutes of this breathing once a day.

Eliminate all caffeine, alcohol, and nicotine from the start (this will help with sleeping better and is, of course, important for baby's health in general).

It's worth noting that although light-exposure therapy is a popular technique, there have been short-term side effects recorded, such as headaches and, ironically, insomnia. You can also just try locking in your bedtime and waking-up time in order to maintain a stable sleep-wake rhythm.

Acupuncture is quite conducive for helping with pregnancy-related sleep disruption by relaxing the nervous system and promoting gentle endorphin production. We also say in Chinese medicine that the mind is stored in the heart. So, by using Chinese medical theory applied to acupuncture points, acupuncture can address the mixed, heart-based emotions that can be coming up during this time in order to quiet the mind. Try the acupressure point (Pericardium 6), which is described in the morning sickness section of this book, on yourself too.

A journal can be a welcome forum for those active pregnancy dreams, or to help an overactive mind relieve looping thoughts.

A snack before bed can also prevent you from hunger in the middle of the night.

Sweet dreams!

pregnancy and can elevate from gas to constipation and heartburn, but staying on the move can help everything move along.

Breast Changes

Breast changes are often among the first indications of pregnancy, and enlargement usually starts to accompany tenderness about eight weeks in, although, in subsequent pregnancies, breasts sometimes don't get as tender or as enlarged because they have been desensitized to the hormone changes from the previous pregnancy.

Normal accompaniments to these changes may include itchiness, stretch marks, and a darkening of your nipples and areolas, along with the bumps on your areolas (Montgomery's tubercles) becoming more noticeable as they start expressing colostrum (a fluid that comes before milk) toward the end of pregnancy.

Va-va-voom! Don't touch me! may be one of the conflicting sentiments as your breasts start to enlarge. In one study, changes in breast size were associated with the baby's gender. Mothers of females developed more pronounced breast changes than mothers of males. This study went on to suggest that from an evolutionary perspective, early breast enlargement in women might function, as it does in other animals, as a sexual stimulus to maintain attractiveness during pregnancy. Considering the many preferences and aspects of attraction, who knows about this, but if the size increase is piquing your partner's interest, it is, alas, usually a taunt, since your breasts are so sore that they're likely off limits.

NOTE: When you're changing up bra sizes, which I recommend doing right away, be sure to stay away from underwire, which can be restrictive to the important flow of blood to your breasts.

Frequent Urination

On another fluid note, the urge to pee can be an early indicator of pregnancy. Contributing factors include hormone changes and increased blood flow to your kidneys, which govern your bladder function. Down the road, this symptom is also exacerbated by the actual pressure of baby growing and compressing your bladder. So, start memorizing all of the bathrooms on your daily routes, but don't let it discourage you from staying extremely

Flatulence: How to Not Fuel the Fire?

Most flatulence is produced from bacteria in the large intestine breaking down food. To assist this process, you can boost up on healthy gut bacteria (see the probiotics recipes throughout this book) and also experiment with eliminating foods that may be culprits for you, such as:

- Fats and dairy products (for a calcium-rich milk alternative, you can try the almond milk recipe, page 32)

- Beans

- Cruciferous veggies such as cabbage, cauliflower, Brussels sprouts, and broccoli

- Asparagus

- Highly processed foods—especially if they have high-fructose corn syrup

- Wheat

- Corn

- Potatoes

- Fried foods

Other tips for lessening intestinal woes are to eat small meals throughout the day, chew really well, drink beverages separately from food, and avoid carbonated drinks—you don't need more things bubbling. A brisk postprandial walk can stimulate your digestion too.

NOTE: Smoking increases stomach acidity. So, if you weren't already motivated to quit smoking, maybe this will put a different kind of fire under you.

hydrated. You can wear a panty liner if you need to account for some extra or unexpected leakage.

Vaginal Bleeding and Cramping

It is always unnerving to see bleeding during your pregnancy. There are obvious connotations. However, bleeding can be normal at different stages, or even throughout a healthy pregnancy. Vaginal bleeding occurs in 15 to 25 percent of early pregnancies, and 50 percent of women who have vaginal bleeding in the first trimester of pregnancy still have a viable pregnancy. Having said that, it's always advisable to get evaluated by your physician to rule out anything else that may be going on—and for your peace of mind.

Always act on the conservative side with bleeding: put your feet up and eat nutritious, iron-rich foods (see the section on anemia, page 137) to help keep up your stamina during this time of not only carrying a baby, but also losing blood.

With first-trimester bleeding, the most common things your physician will be working to rule out are miscarriage, ectopic pregnancy, cervical infections (which can inflame and agitate your vaginal tissue), and gestational trophoblastic disease (a very rare pregnancy-related tumor).

I've seen women go through entire pregnancies with what resembles a level of bleeding that you might associate with your period, and still have wonderfully healthy babies.

The first step to identifying the cause of the bleeding is to talk to your healthcare provider, but here are some tips for beginning to interpret the data for what's typically within a safe, albeit disconcerting zone:

- Spotting and light bleeding episodes are not typically a risk for miscarriage, especially if the bleeding lasts for only one to two days.

- Heavy bleeding in the first trimester, especially when there's also pain, is associated with higher risk of miscarriage.

- Seeing the yolk sac within the gestational sac during an ultrasound is a definitive sign of a healthy beginning to pregnancy, regardless of bleeding.

Cramping that feels like menstrual twinges often accompanies spotting and can be indicative of implantation, which occurs approximately seven to ten days after ovulation. As the baby continues to settle in to his or her new home in your endometrial lining, this periodic cramping might continue. This is different than sharp, stabbing, continual, and localized pain, which warrants getting checked out.

A Note on Miscarriage

Miscarriage is, of course, one of a pregnant woman's earliest and most pro-found concerns. In the unlikely event you suffer a miscarriage, I can confi-dently say that there's nothing you did to cause your pregnancy loss. It is very hard to disrupt a viable pregnancy.

Unfortunately, miscarriage occurs as a normal part reproductive life for many women—and it doesn't mean anything about your ability to successfully carry your next child. As a matter of fact, it's not until three pregnancy losses occur that most doctors recommend evaluation, and even then, 70 percent of pregnancies after recurrent losses have a chance of success. This is certainly not meant to make you worry about miscarriage, nor to diminish the severity or grief that you may experience in the event of a miscarriage, but some-times, having the facts under your belt can provide an avenue of hope.

In the case of possible genetic abnormalities, which is the most prevalent thought around the cause of otherwise unknown reasons in a pregnancy loss—especially as one ages, nature usually makes the tough decision for you, but if you feel inclined to investigate the cause of your miscarriage, you can consult with a gynecologist or reproductive endocrinologist for a tissue biopsy and investigate what may have happened, plus add some strategies that may prepare you to try again with more success.

I also encourage you to seek out resources such as therapists or books on pregnancy loss, and some physical support such as acupuncture or massage, during this difficult time to help you gain insight and heal.

Cancer in Pregnancy

The most common cancers in pregnancy are estrogen-sensitive cancers such as breast (there's even a specific diagnosis called pregnancy-associated breast cancer) and cervical. There are now a multitude of ways to safely diagnose and begin to address these cancers during pregnancy. Although it is a daunt-ing diagnosis and can impose on breastfeeding (if receiving chemotherapy or radiation after delivery the drugs pass through the milk, and the process itself may diminish your milk supply), cancer itself rarely harms the baby.

Treatment decision should be made collaboratively with a multidisciplinary team including your gynecologist, oncologist, and a pediatrician.

Molar Pregnancy and Choriocarcinomas

A hydatidiform mole (also called a molar pregnancy) occurs when sperm cells fertilize an egg that doesn't contain a nucleus (the mother's DNA). So, all the genetic material is from the sperm cell, which of course precludes the possibility of a baby being able to form. Surgery is the solution. However, the abnormal tissue of the mole can continue to grow after surgery, which is the primary contributing factor to choriocarcinoma.

Choriocarcinoma is a rare, malignant cancer of the uterus that most often occurs after a hydatidiform mole but can also arise from a miscarriage, tubal pregnancy, or even a normal previous pregnancy. This cancer is classified as a gestational trophoblastic disease (GTD).

Trophoblasts are cells on the outer layer of a blastocyst, which provide nutrients to the embryo and develop into the placenta, but in this condition, the cells grow into the lining of the uterus. This is a more complex condition that will require your specialists to get on board to navigate a treatment path.

Bell's Palsy

Bell's palsy is characterized by one-sided weakness or paralysis of the face and often discomfort on one side of your head. It comes on suddenly and usually gets worse over a period of a few days. Thirty percent of the time, Bell's palsy can be a predictor for preeclampsia.

Although you might feel temporarily disfigured, this is a beautiful example of how Chinese medicine can give insight into origins and relationships of a symptom for a Western diagnosis that doesn't have a known reason or good treatment strategy. The Chinese medicine explanation (you'll definitely have to step out of your Western mind for a moment for this) is that when the Liver, which is very active during pregnancy (it governs important aspects of reproduction, hormones and processing stress), gets a bit enraged (usually from an encounter with stress) it generates heat, and just like heat rises, the Liver "flares" up and drives these internal symptoms to the head and face. This is called "Liver wind."

The very real result of this euphemistic "Liver wind," is Bell's palsy. This is also the same mechanism that causes high blood pressure. So, from a Chinese medicine model, it makes perfect sense that Bell's palsy and high blood pressure (an aspect of preeclampsia) go together. The good news is that acupuncture can target the Liver system to get things back in check. So, see an acupuncturist for this one—the sooner the better, as results for this are more reliable if you can expedite your treatment.

As a side note, if you have an incidence of Bell's palsy, you might need to rule out Lyme disease, as Bell's can be a symptom of that tricky-to-diagnose condition.

Epilepsy

Epilepsy and other seizure-related disorders can be unpredictable and dangerous during pregnancy if not managed with appropriate medications. This is very challenging, since adverse outcomes during pregnancy, such as congenital malformations, are associated with antiepileptic drugs. Additionally, estrogen, which is at an all-time high during pregnancy, has been shown to lower your seizure threshold (making you more susceptible). Perhaps to balance this, progesterone, which is also dominant in pregnancy, has an anti-seizure effect, but our bodies don't necessarily provide us with all of the management or balance that we need.

Our body can, however, hint at our potential well-being. Studies have shown that epileptic women who are free from seizures for one full year before pregnancy are less likely to suffer from seizures during pregnancy. If you suffer from epilepsy, the best strategy for pregnancy is to assess your current medication levels with your physician and receive close monitoring throughout your pregnancy.

In Chinese medicine, epilepsy is attributed to a more extreme gradient of the "Liver wind" that we discussed in the Bell's palsy section above, and just as with Bell's palsy, acupuncture can be a safe and viable method for managing and treating seizure disorders.

NOTE: A standard supplement recommendation for pregnant women with epilepsy is to take 5 milligrams of folic acid daily.

Metallic Taste

The technical name for the metallic taste you might experience before you even know you're pregnant is called *dysgeusia*, which you might notice sounds an awful lot like "disgusting." Dysgeusia isn't limited to the flavor of pennies corroding in your mouth; you might also notice a sour or bitter flavor.

Dysgeusia comes from the same origins as nausea and vomiting—which is to say, we don't really know why it happens from a Western point of view. Although, we can surmise that the notable changes in the secretion of hormones that occurs during this stage may be partially responsible. Chinese medicine relates sour and bitter flavor profiles to the action of the Liver, which as you now know, is an active system during this time, and women who experience severe nausea and vomiting (also a Liver-driven theme) tend to be the ones who also experience dysgeusia.

It's also common to develop an enhanced sense of smell during pregnancy, which is intimately connected to your sense of taste. Like nausea and vomiting, dysgeusia typically recedes or disappears altogether in the second trimester.

In the meantime, to troubleshoot:

- Assess your current medications (some medications can cause a metallic taste).
- Make sure you're taking your prenatal vitamin to get enough B12 and zinc, as those deficiencies can be a potential source of the metallic taste.
- Check out your oral health with your dentist (and be sure they're well-versed in preganacy-safe dentistry modifications).
- Drink the Morning Mocktail recipe—it might help override the unpleasant taste as well as strengthen your digestion.
- Concoct and swish with the recipes for Mild Mouthwash or Green Tea Mouthwash on pages 27–28.

....

MORNING MOCKTAIL

In addition to being very hydrating, this drink is rich in magnesium, fiber, and enzymes and is a good source of beneficial fats and oils. It's also an efficient way to get a full spectrum of green veggies into your diet if you're not inclined to be eating a pile of them every day. As you may recall, green is also the color that's associated with the Liver system. So, boosting up on these greens means a boost to this whole system.

Put a handful of each or some (depending on availability and inclination) of the following veggies in a blender, with equal parts coconut water and coconut milk to mask the "greenness" a bit and increase electrolytes and subsequent hydration.

Celery

Beet greens

Dandelion greens

Parsley

Cilantro

Swiss chard

Kale

Pineapple chunks

A small piece of chopped ginger root (optional based on discussion of herbal teas in the beginning of this section)

1 tablespoon coconut oil

Strain through fine mesh if your blender doesn't liquefy the ingredients.

....

MILD MOUTHWASH

Mix ¼ teaspoon baking soda in 8 ounces of water and swish and spit to neutralize the pH levels in your mouth.

....

....

GREEN TEA MOUTHWASH

1 teaspoon powdered green tea (also known as Matcha)

Dissolve and mix the powder in warm water and swish and spit to enhance antibacterial and anti-inflammatory activity in your mouth. See resource section for where to get powdered green tea.

....

Rhesus Factor (Rh Factor)

None of us likes the idea of outright rejecting our offspring, but sometimes our body doesn't cooperate with our feelings. Rhesus Factor (Rh) can be one of those times. Rh is a protein on the surface of red blood cells. If you have this protein, you are Rh positive, and if you don't, you're Rh negative.

If you're Rh negative and your baby is Rh positive, your body might produce antibodies that attack baby's red blood cells. This only becomes relevant during pregnancy (and is kind of like an allergic reaction to bee stings, which gets much worse with the second sting—in other words, it is often only an issue in subsequent pregnancies). And since your baby has its own blood system during the pregnancy, it is really only relevant during delivery, amniocentesis, or chorionic villus sampling—when your blood can comingle with baby's.

If you're Rh negative, you'll be monitored through blood tests at different stages during your pregnancy, and you may be required to get an injection of Rh immune globulin to help prevent your body from producing Rh antibodies. If you're already producing these antibodies, the injection won't counteract it. You and baby will be monitored for the possibility of baby needing a blood transfusion either during pregnancy (through the umbilical cord) or right after birth.

It's helpful to get dad measured for Rh factor too, because if you're negative and he's negative, baby will always be negative, but if you're negative and dad is positive, you have the unknown variable of baby possibly being either Rh positive or Rh negative.

The Basic Prenatal Checkup Schedule

Your checkups can range from making you feel comforted to overly monitored. Since much of pregnancy is just like parenthood, navigating on your own the best you can in-between visits may console you. Having said that, there are plenty of studies that indicate regular checkups produce healthier babies. We can deduce that this helps everyone catch any issues as soon as possible. However, visit increments vary depending on your needs, desires, and the advice of your practitioner. And note that there is usually an increased frequency of visits if you are carrying multiples. Here are some general guidelines for what to expect:

Four to twenty-eight weeks
One visit per month

Twenty-eight to thirty-six weeks
Two visits per month

Thirty-six weeks to delivery
One visit per week

Living with Your Liver

Some liver conditions such as HELLP syndrome are unique to pregnancy, but others such as hepatitis may be pre-existing issues. Either way, optimizing your liver's function during pregnancy is an important aspect of managing your care.

HELLP Syndrome

HELLP is an acronym for hemolysis, elevated liver enzymes, and low platelet-count syndrome. Thankfully, the occurrence of this pathology is small (happening in only about 0.8 percent of pregnancies), but this risk increases to 10 percent if you have severe preeclampsia, which is really the only thing to monitor, since there are rarely any hints at the acute

Exercise

The analysis of available research on exercise and pregnancy basically says to do what you did before—unless you did nothing before you got pregnant, or are prone to running marathons regularly. Essentially, you should continue to exercise moderately and mindfully. You are your own best barometer for what's right for your body during this time. Exercise has many health benefits, such as endorphins and cardiovascular strengthening that can contribute to your pregnancy and your own health and well-being during pregnancy.

A general guideline to keeping your heart rate within good boundaries is to still be able to talk while you're exercising. I also recommend avoiding extremely heavy lifting or severe abdominal crunching. Although, the truth is, it's very hard to dislodge a viable pregnancy. Babies are resilient, and so are you.

Some pregnancy-conducive exercises to explore, if you haven't already, are prenatal-specific yoga and Pilates. Both emphasize relaxation and strengthening. Swimming is wonderful for building lung capacity and counteracting shortness of breath, and walking and hiking are great for circulation and bone density. Just be aware of how the hormone relaxin can leave your ligaments a little looser and predispose you to sprains and strains with rigorous, weight-bearing exercise. So, make sure to stretch, and no matter what you do, always pay close attention and be responsive to your body's needs and sensations.

development of HELLP. If this syndrome develops, it is a severe and potentially life-threatening issue that needs immediate emergency medical intervention.

Hepatitis

The word *hepatitis* translates from its Greek and Latin roots to literally mean "inflammation of the liver," and the ABCs of this inflammatory process of the largest internal organ (the skin being the largest organ overall) actually include hepatitis A, B, C, D, E, G, and X. However, the most prevalent ones that we're concerned with are A, B, and C.

The Truth about Caffeine

We're all entitled to a vice, and coffee is a worldwide choice. It's actually the number one source of antioxidants for most people. During pregnancy, however, it's time to let it go. Caffeine is not evil, but in pregnancy its role is controversial, and there is enough evidence that points to it being unfavorable—especially in early pregnancy. When we talk about caffeine, we're not just talking about coffee but also caffeinated teas, soda, and some over-the-counter medications.

Western medical literature does say that drinking one to three cups of coffee per day is okay, but caffeine stays in a pregnant woman's system for about triple the amount of time that it circulates in a nonpregnant woman, and to boot, it crosses the placental barrier, where the baby lacks the adult enzyme needed to effectively metabolize the caffeine. Since caffeine has been linked with low birth weight, preterm delivery, and even miscarriage, I say try another method of indulgence for these ten months (and a bit more, if you're breastfeeding). After all, research indicates that adrenaline doesn't even come from the coffee itself, but from the anticipation of the cup of coffee. So, maybe you can rewire your excitement into a cup of hot cocoa.

Chocolate, contrary to popular belief, does not contain the same stimulant as coffee. Chocolate contains an alkaloid called theobromine, which is in the same class of compounds as caffeine, but is not caffeine. However, since they're related, chocolate should also be consumed in moderation for some of the same reasons. If you need a little indulgence, the benefits of a cup of cocoa do outweigh the potential negative side effects of coffee. Chocolate, with a 70 percent cacao content, has been shown to contribute to reducing blood pressure and stabilizing blood sugar during pregnancy and may lower the risk of preeclampsia.

A Note on Decaffeinated Coffee

Although it initially seems like a better option, if it's not water processed, that means harsher chemicals are used to filter out the caffeine—also not good for you or baby. Even decaf has a little bit of caffeine in it, and with the extended stay of caffeine in your body during pregnancy, it's just not the best choice.

···

COFFEE ALTERNATIVE:
COCOA WITH HOMEMADE ALMOND MILK

Cocoa Ingredients

½ part carob powder (found at most health-food stores, and of course online)

½ part cocoa powder (70 percent cacao content)

Almond Milk Ingredients

1 cup raw, unsalted almonds, skin-on

4 cups filtered water, plus more water for soaking almonds

1 ½ teaspoons honey, or one whole pitted date

Dash of salt

You will also need

Blender

Fine mesh strainer or muslin cloth

1-quart glass jar or storage container

Directions

Blend all of the almond milk ingredients together on high until liquefied, and strain into your jar or storage container. Pour 1 cup of almond milk into a small saucepan and keep the rest in the fridge for next time. Bring almond milk to a simmer and slowly add carob and cocoa powder to taste. I recommend starting with 1 tablespoon of each. Continue to stir or whisk until thoroughly blended and warm.

···

Hepatitis A (HAV)

HAV is contracted from contaminated food, water, or feces. Pretty much everyone who develops HAV makes a spontaneous, full recovery without the need for intervention and without running the risk of developing a chronic liver condition. If your baby is exposed, the infection is usually mild and the good news is that the baby will have immunity to it for life, but you can minimize your chances of getting HAV by managing your sanitation—washing your hands and your food. The main treatment is rest and a nutritious diet.

Hepatitis B (HBV)

HBV is transmitted through infected body fluids such as blood (which is the primary way that your baby is potentially affected during birth), sexual fluids, or from being pricked by an unsterilized needle. It is inconclusive whether or not C-section mitigates the risk of transmission to your baby, and although HBV is also transmitted through breast milk, when you're not on antiviral therapy; if your baby is vaccinated, breastfeeding is not contraindicated.

Treatment strategies such as the antiviral medication Tenofovir (Viread) depend on your viral load and how advanced your condition is. As ever, managing anything during pregnancy includes balancing an analysis of the risks and benefits to you and baby.

To be up-to-date on taking antivirals for HBV during pregnancy, you can check out the antiretroviral pregnancy registry (APR): http://www .apregis try. com/forms/interim_report.pdf.

Preventing HBV includes practicing safe sex and not sharing any personal items that can impart traces of blood such as razors or manicure implements. For managing HBV during pregnancy, rest and nutrition geared around repairing the liver are essential. The basic nutritional principles are to eat low-fat, easy-to-digest foods such as broths and soups with lots of bitter greens such as dandelion, chicory, and endives (these help stimulate the liver to process bile and eliminate toxins more effectively), and spices that are known to contain liver-protecting compounds, including turmeric, garlic, and black pepper.

Additionally, start each morning with a glass of warm water with half of a freshly squeezed lemon in it (helps the liver to gently flush out accumulations.) Continue to hydrate throughout the day with electrolyte drinks (see the Electrolyte Refresher recipe on page 37 to make your own), and incorporate some of the supplements below.

Hepatitis C (HCV)

HCV is usually spread through direct contact with HCV-infected blood. The approaches to prevention and management are similar to HBV, but there's not a safe medication treatment available during pregnancy.

Some pregnancy-safe support to boost immunity during pregnancy can include:

- Vitamin C: 1,000 mg one to three times a day (antioxidant)
- Co Enzyme Q10: 200 mg at night (antioxidant)
- Acetyl-L-carnitine: 500 mg a day (antiviral and antioxidant)
- Probiotics containing *Lactobacillus acidophilus* (if you are taking immune-suppressive drugs, only take under supervision)
- N-acetyl cysteine (NAC): 200-500 mg three times a day (liver and antioxidant support)
- Cordyceps: 3 grams two times a day (a Chinese medicinal mushroom to support the liver and improve the immune system)
- Reishi mushroom: 150-300 mg two times a day (another type of mushroom used in traditional Chinese medicine to decrease the hepatitis virus)

Supplements and medications to avoid because they are particularly harsh on the liver include:

- Vitamin A
- Tylenol

Acute Fatty Liver

The causes of this pregnancy-specific condition aren't always known, but if the liver already has scar tissue or cirrhosis from chronic hepatitis, the extra demands on this organ during pregnancy may predispose you to this condition. It's also postulated that acute fatty liver can arise from a deficiency of an enzyme produced by the liver that normally allows pregnant women to metabolize fatty acids.

Symptoms are most common during the third trimester: nausea, vomiting, pain in your upper abdomen, jaundice, and increased thirst and urination. This condition can become incredibly severe fairly quickly and can adversely affect both you and your baby. Your baby could be born with a deficiency in this enzyme, but the more severe threat is a high mortality rate for such pregnancies. The only treatment is a delivery at the earliest time that's relatively safe, typically followed by plasma-exchange therapy. Barring severe damage, there's a good prognosis for recovery for everyone after birth.

Anatomy of a Prenatal Vitamin

Pregnancy is an amazing time of change in your body and in your life. It's important to take prenatal supplements, but note the word "supplement"—prenatals are not intended to replace the nutrition you get from food, but to round it out. They should be used with a backdrop of striving for good nutrition through whole foods. The foods you eat before and during your pregnancy will prepare your body to support healthy growth and development and contribute to a nourished pregnancy and birth.

During this time, you need extra food and nutrients. Here's a review, based on the Dietary Reference Intake (DRI) from the Institute of Medicine (IOM) of what a pregnant woman should consume and how much. You can use this information to inform you about attaining optimum health for you and your baby's growing needs and as a guide for assessing a prenatal vitamin and incorporating the appropriate foods alongside your vitamins.

If you're worried that you're not getting enough of something, it can be easy to duplicate nutrients by taking them through multiple supplements. But keep in mind that there can be too much of a good thing. So, be sure to refer to the guidelines on the upper limit (UL) of certain nutrients that you don't want to take too much of.

As a foundation for your prenatal vitamin support, a couple of high quality brands that I recommend, which are typically easier to get down than some of the others, are an over the counter option such as Rainbow Light (see resource section) and Thorne, which you can get prescribed through your healthcare provider.

NOTE: I recommend avoiding prenatal vitamins with fish oil in them. Fish oil can easily go rancid and corrupt the health-giving effects of the other nutrients—rendering them more harmful than helpful. If you're taking fish oil, be sure to source a brand that is refrigerated and screened well for heavy metals, toxins, and other contaminants.

The Fundamental Building Blocks for Your Daily Nutrition

Calories: 2,300-3,200 (if you're carrying multiples, add 300 calories more for each additional baby)

Fiber: 28 grams

Protein: 71 grams (increase about 10 grams per trimester)

Carbohydrates: 175 grams

Water: 3 liters

VITAMIN A 770 MCG (UL 3,000 MCG)

Also known as Retinol, vitamin A is important for the development of the heart, lungs, kidneys, eyes, and bones, as well as the circulatory, respiratory, and central nervous system. It also helps with resistance to infection and aids fat metabolism and helps maintain normal vision. Vitamin A is particularly essential for women who are about to give birth, because it helps with postpartum tissue repair.

Having said all of that, too much vitamin A can cause birth defects. 770 mcg or the equivalent, 2,565 international units (IU) of vitamin A is the daily recommended dose for pregnant women. For perspective, three ounces of cooked beef liver contains 27,185 IU and three ounces of cooked chicken liver contains 12,325 IU. The food sources of vitamin A below will help you define what to include in your diet so as not to be too intimidated by this important nutrient.

Food Sources: Vitamin A from animal sources such as beef, liver, and cod liver oil is fat soluble and can build up and become toxic, whereas plant or carotenoid sources do not accumulate in the body in the same way. So, foods such as butternut squash, cantaloupe, carrots, dried apricots, kale, papayas, paprika, peaches, pumpkins, spinach, sweet potatoes, and turnips are preferable sources of vitamin A during pregnancy.

VITAMIN C (AS ASCORBIC ACID) 150 MG (UL 2,000 MG)

Vitamin C contributes to tissue repair, specifically the production of collagen—a structural component of cartilage, tendons, bones, and skin. It is also

....

VITAMIN C-RICH ELECTROLYTE REFRESHER

This electrolyte beverage can help you boost up on vitamin C and keep you hydrated by transporting fluids and nutrients to your cells. Here's how to make your own delicious, low-sugar electrolyte drink:

Ingredients

Water

Coconut Water

Sea Salt

Citrus Juice (mix and match orange, grapefruit, lemon, lime to your liking). Fresh squeezed has the highest degree of nutrients and is always the most delicious, but it's fine to use store bought in a pinch.

Coconut Sugar or Honey (optional)

Directions

Mix equal parts water and coconut water (which has natural electrolytes in it). Add a pinch of sea salt (even though this increases fluid retention, it also helps with fluid transportation). Squeeze in citrus juice from oranges, grapefruits, lemons, or limes. Add an optional small amount of organic coconut sugar or honey.

You can keep a jug of this refresher in the fridge to sip on.

....

an antioxidant that protects you from cellular damage, aids your body in fighting infections, and helps you absorb iron.

Food Sources: Citrus fruits, broccoli, cabbage, green peppers, melons, oranges, potatoes, strawberries, and tomatoes.

CALCIUM (AS CALCIUM CITRATE-MALATE) 1,000 MG (UL 2,500 MG)
As a culture, our current calcium intake is about a quarter of what we used to consume before the start of agriculture about 10,000 years ago. So, most of us run a little calcium deficient, and the need for calcium is even 50 percent greater during pregnancy.

Calcium helps form the baby's teeth and bones, aids in heart and muscle function, and is important for blood clotting and proper nerve function. If you don't have enough calcium, your body will pull it from your bones, and since the minerals in the body are in a delicate, dynamic balance, if a deficiency in calcium exists, other minerals may also be out of balance. The following recommendations to increase calcium absorption should also improve the effective utilization of all minerals in the body.

Food Sources: Contrary to popular belief, calcium from milk sources is usually not well absorbed or tolerated. Some high-quality yogurts and kefirs contain probiotics and pose an exception to this rule. In general, more easily assimilated calcium-rich pregnancy foods include:

- Arugula
- Beans (adzuki, black, lima, mung, soybeans)
- Blackstrap molasses
- Chicken
- Collard greens
- Dark chocolate (high-quality and at least 70 percent cacao content)
- Dried fruit (figs, prunes)
- Dried seaweeds (arame, hijiki, kelp, kombu, wakame)
- High-chlorophyll foods (blue-green algae, chlorella, spirulina, wheat or barley grass)
- Kale
- Nuts and seeds (almonds, cashews, hazelnuts, sesame seeds)
- Parsley
- Pumpkin
- Quinoa
- Sardines
- Tofu
- Turnip greens
- Watercress
- Whole grains (barley, buckwheat, corn, millet, rice, rye, wheat berries)

NOTE: Some sea vegetables provide ten times as much calcium as cow's milk, and three cups of arugula (basically a full salad portion) provide 400 mg of calcium.

Just as it's important to get enough calcium from the foods you eat, it's also important to avoid foods and substances that inhibit the absorption of calcium.

Foods and substances that inhibit calcium absorption:

- Alcohol
- Cigarettes
- Coffee
- Diuretics
- Excessive protein
- Excessive salt
- Refined sugar
- Soft drinks
- Bell peppers, eggplant, potatoes, and tomatoes (these vegetables contain the calcium inhibitor solanine)
- Too little or too much exercise (moderate exercise prevents calcium loss, but excessive physical activity has been shown to cause calcium loss)

VITAMIN D (AS VITAMIN D3) 5,000 IU IN EARLY PREGNANCY AND 6,000 IU IN LATER STAGES (UL 10,000 IU)

Without the pre-hormone vitamin D, we do not have the substrate for calcitriol (the hormonally active form of vitamin D), which is pivotal for brain development—especially during pregnancy. Vitamin D also helps your body maintain proper levels of calcium and phosphorous to build your baby's bones and teeth.

A vitamin D deficiency during pregnancy can cause slowed growth and skeletal deformities and may also have an impact on increased risk for rickets in babies, low birth weight, delayed development, and long-term lowered immune function. A deficiency of vitamin D has also been linked to a greater risk of pregnancy complications, including preeclampsia.

CALCIUM-RICH SEA VEGETABLE QUINOA BOWL
Makes 4 servings

Ingredients

1 cup dried quinoa

3 cups water or vegetable or chicken stock (see Boosted-Up Chicken Stock recipe)

1 cup kale, finely chopped

¼ cup basil, coarsely chopped

2 tablespoons nutritional yeast

1 tablespoon dulse flakes (a sea vegetable that can be found in many health or specialty food stores)

½ a lemon, juiced

½ an avocado

1 tablespoon flax seeds

1 tablespoon pumpkin seeds

2 tablespoons cold-pressed olive oil

A pinch of sea salt

Directions

Rinse quinoa and drain. Bring quinoa and water or stock to a boil. When the water boils, reduce to a simmer. Simmer with lid not completely on, allowing some air to escape.

Cook for about twenty minutes, or until the liquid has evaporated and the quinoa is cooked.

Stir in the kale, basil, nutritional yeast, dulse flakes, and lemon juice. Top with avocado, flax, and pumpkin seeds. Drizzle olive oil over the top and season with sea salt.

CALCIUM-RICH SAVORY MEDITERRANEAN YOGURT

This dish is a nice change of pace that incorporates both sweet and savory flavors. Chickpeas (garbanzo beans) are an incredible source of folate as well.

Ingredients

¼ cup finely chopped yellow onion

2 tablespoons butter or ghee (clarified butter)

1 large garlic clove, minced

½ teaspoon ground cumin

A pinch of ground turmeric

One 15-ounce, BPA-free can of chickpeas, drained (or cooked from dried chickpeas)

1 cup water or chicken or vegetable broth

Lemon wedge

Salt and freshly ground black pepper, to taste

¼ cup slivered almonds and/or walnuts

1 ½ cups whole-fat yogurt with live cultures

1 cup chopped or grated cucumber

1 tablespoon chopped mint

Directions

In a medium skillet, heat the butter or ghee until it melts but does not brown.

Add onion and garlic and cook over medium heat until onion is translucent, five to seven minutes.

Stir in cumin and turmeric, stirring, for one minute. Add the chickpeas and broth and bring to a boil. Cover and simmer over low heat for fifteen minutes. Remove lid and bring back to a boil. Cook, uncovered, until the liquid is reduced, about three minutes. Stir in a squeeze of lemon and season with salt and pepper. In a small, dry skillet, toast the almonds or walnuts, stirring, until golden—about four minutes. Scoop yogurt into a bowl and top with chickpea mixture, nuts, cucumber, and mint.

Food and Lifestyle Sources: Vitamin D isn't actually a vitamin at all. It's a prehormone that is catalyzed into useable vitamin D by a heat reaction, which may account for part of the reason that sun exposure is necessary for vitamin D conversion. Vitamin D can be obtained through dietary intake, but unless you have a diet rich in reindeer meat, lichen, or seagull eggs, it is unlikely that you are getting adequate dietary sources. So, make sure you get some sun, and since prenatal vitamins usually only contain a trace level of vitamin D, supplement with a liquid form of vitamin D as well.

FOLIC ACID AND FOLATE (AS 5-METHYLTETRAHYDROFOLATE) 600 MCG (UL 1,000 MCG)

These two terms for vitamin B9 are often used interchangeably, but folate occurs naturally in food and folic acid is the synthetic compound. The body tends to metabolize the food source better, and since this is such an essential ingredient for pregnancy for helping to prevent neural tube defects (NTDs)—serious birth defects of the spinal cord (such as spina bifida) and the brain—it's ideal to be getting your dose in even before you conceive, but certainly throughout pregnancy. Some research suggests that getting enough folate may also help lower your baby's risk of other defects such as cleft lip, cleft palate, and certain types of heart abnormalities.

Your body also requires folate to make normal red blood cells and prevent anemia, and it's essential for the production, repair, and function of basic cellular building blocks. So, getting enough folate is particularly important for you and the rapid cell growth of your placenta and developing baby.

Food and Supplement Sources: To boost your supplementation, good food sources of folate are: asparagus, broccoli, chicken liver (just be mindful of the amount of this one based on the vitamin A discussion), dark leafy greens, dried peas and beans, green beans, green peas, melons, oranges, spinach, and turnip greens.

NOTE: If using a supplement, look for methylated folate (called 5-MTHF). Unlike folic acid, it doesn't need to be converted by the liver. So it delivers the usable folate directly to your system and doesn't mask B12 deficiency.

IRON (AS IRON PICOLINATE) 27 MG (UL 45 MG)

Iron is recommended to help prevent or treat anemia and helps the placenta develop and keeps you and your baby strong.

....

IRON WOMAN ENERGY SNACKS

Put all of the following in a mixing bowl, stir, and shape into bite-sized morsels to keep in the fridge and snack on one to two times a day:

½ cup tahini (sesame seed butter)

½ cup almond butter

2 tablespoons molasses

1 tablespoon wheat germ (take out if you eat gluten free)

1 tablespoon ground flax seeds

1 teaspoon spirulina or other green, chlorophyll-based powder\

....

Food Sources: There are two types of iron that you get from food: *heme* and *nonheme*. Heme iron is found in animal foods such as egg yolks, poultry, liver, red meat, salmon, and sardines canned in oil; nonheme iron comes from plant sources such as artichokes, baked potatoes, beets, broccoli, chickpeas, dried apricots, dried prunes, figs, lentils, lima beans, molasses, oatmeal, pumpkin seeds, sesame seeds, and wheat germ.

NOTE: Plant-based irons are best absorbed if eaten with foods rich in vitamin C such as dark leafy greens (kale, mustard greens, Swiss chard etc.), papaya, parsley, and thyme. Iron absorption from any source is interfered with when consumed with tea or coffee.

THIAMIN (AS THIAMIN HCL) 4 MG

Also known as vitamin B1, thiamin enables you and your baby to convert carbohydrates into energy. It's essential for your baby's brain development and aids the normal functioning of your nervous system, muscles, and heart.

Food Sources: Thiamin is found in brown rice, flax seeds, legumes, oatmeal, potatoes (skin on), sunflower seeds, and watermelon.

RIBOFLAVIN (AS RIBOFLAVIN 5-PHOSPHATE SODIUM) 3.6 MG

Also known as vitamin B2, riboflavin helps your body produce energy. It promotes growth, vision, and healthy skin, and it's important for your baby's bone, muscle, and nerve development. Riboflavin is a water-soluble vitamin, which means your body doesn't store it, so you'll need to consume enough each day.

Food Sources: Riboflavin is found in soybeans, beet greens, yogurt, spinach, eggs, and almonds.

VITAMIN B6 (AS PYRIDOXAL 5-PHOSPHATE) 10 MG (UL 100 MG)

Also known as pyridoxine, B6 helps your body metabolize protein, fats, and carbohydrates. It also helps form new red blood cells, antibodies, and neurotransmitters and is vital to your baby's developing brain and nervous system.

....

IRON-RICH KALE CHIPS

Chop a bunch of destemmed kale into about 3-inch pieces and lightly coat with olive oil and mustard. Spread on a lined baking sheet and cook in a preheated oven at 350 for approximately twenty minutes. NOTE: Kale should be allowed to dry thoroughly after rinsing, or it won't get crispy.

....

PUMPKIN SEED PESTO

This is a delicious and iron-rich spread you can eat on crackers or bread, use as a vegetable dip, mash with a sweet yam, or add to pasta. In a food processor or blender, pulse the following ingredients:

6 tablespoons extra-virgin olive oil (you can use more or less depending on your texture preference)

A handful of fresh herbs such as basil, cilantro, and parsley

1 tablespoon tahini butter

1 tablespoon pumpkin seeds

2 tablespoons of walnuts and/or pine nuts

A dash of salt

1 clove of fresh garlic (omit if you're having digestive trouble)

....

NOTE: Research shows that extra vitamin B6 may relieve nausea and vomiting for some women during pregnancy. See section on morning sickness for more info on using B6 for nausea and vomiting.

Food Sources: Vitamin B6 is found most prevalently in bananas, beef, salmon, and sunflower seeds.

ADDITIONAL NUTRIENTS

In addition to the above crucial elements, a good prenatal vitamin will also contain:

Niacin (as niacinamide) 30 mg (UL 35 mg)

Vitamin E (as d-alpha tocopheryl) 15 mg (UL 1,000 mg)

Vitamin K (as vitamin K1) 100 mcg

Vitamin B12 (100 mcg as adenosylcobalamin and 100 mcg as methylcobalamin) 200 mcg

Biotin 50 mcg

Pantothenic Acid (as calcium panothenate) 16 mg

Iodine (as potassium iodide) 150 mcg (1,100 mcg)

Magnesium (as magnesium citrate-malate) 100 mg (UL 350 mg)

Zinc (as zinc picolinate) 25 mg (UL 40 mg)

Selenium (as selenium picolinate) 50 mcg (UL 400 mcg)

Copper (as copper picolinate) 2500 mcg (10,000 mcg)

Manganese (as manganese picolinate) 5 mg (UL 11 mg)

Chromium (as chromium picolinate) 100 mcg

Molybdenum (as molybdenum picolinate) 50 mcg (UL 2,000 mcg)

Boron (as boron picolinate) 1 mg (UL 20 mg)

A Note on Fats and Sugar

Don't be scared of fat. The right types of fat are necessary for proper growth and development of your baby. Good sources of essential fats are avocados; fish (after the first trimester) such as mackerel, salmon, and sardines; flax seeds; nuts such as almonds, hazelnuts, and walnuts; and oils such as coconut oil, olive oil, and sesame oil.

As for sugar, optimizing nutrients isn't just about consuming the right things, but also being attentive to things that leach the precious little sustenance you are likely able to get down right now. Sugar does just that, and should be minimized in order to maximize your other nutrients.

If you're craving sugar, a good way to begin to diminish the craving is to boost up on protein. Instead of a pastry, a great go-to food is a yam or sweet potato, which can satiate your craving for sweets without assaulting your blood sugar. Here are two recipes to keep on hand—a protein-rich soup base and a sweet potato puree.

....

BOOSTED-UP CHICKEN STOCK

Folklore strikes again. A chicken is able to lay an egg pretty much every day, and in Chinese medicine, we encourage you too to replenish daily with this easy to digest, protein-rich broth to help you hatch your healthy baby. As queasiness sets in, it's a great way to consume a gentle-to-digest, mineral-rich food source—and doubles as a base for other recipes that call for stock.

Ingredients

> 1 pound organic chicken or beef bones from your local health-food store or butcher (you can also just put a whole, uncooked chicken in the pot and use the meat for a plethora of dishes)
>
> * As a variation, use 1.5-2 pounds of beef knuckle bones
>
> 3 carrots, scrubbed and chopped
>
> 3 celery stalks, chopped
>
> 2 inches of fresh ginger root, chopped
>
> 1 onion, peeled and halved
>
> 1 lemon, washed and halved
>
> Whole head of fresh garlic, peeled and smashed
>
> Generous tablespoon of sea salt
>
> Water to fill stockpot
>
> 1 bunch parsley, chopped

2 tablespoons apple cider vinegar

1 tablespoon coconut oil

Directions

In a large pot, add the coconut oil and brown the bones on all sides over medium-high heat. Add everything else but the parsley, and fill stockpot almost full with water. Bring to a boil, and then reduce to a simmer for eight hours up to overnight (it will only get richer), periodically skimming the fat off the top. Add parsley, then turn off the heat. Strain the solids out through a colander and discard or reincorporate carrots and celery and chicken pieces (if you've used a whole chicken) into the soup.

The broth can be sipped as-is, or used as a base for other soups and recipes in this book and beyond. If you're not going to use the stock within a few days, freeze it.

....

SWEET POTATO PURÉE

Use the stock in the last recipe as a base to puree ¼ cup of homemade stock with 1 cup steamed sweet potatoes, 1 tablespoon of butter or ghee, and a pinch of cumin. Top with cilantro and a squeeze of lime.

....

Checklist for Month One

- Take your prenatal vitamin.
- Eat like you're taking a prenatal vitamin.
- Familiarize yourself with pregnancy nutrition, including the safe and not-so-safe pregnancy foods.
- No more changing the cat litter.
- Review your health insurance.
- Find an obstetrician and/or midwife, and schedule and prepare for your first prenatal appointment.
- Confirm whether any prescriptions you're currently taking are not safe during pregnancy.

- No more martinis or smoking (See section on How to Quit Smoking in month three).
- Start some preemptive antinausea techniques such the Morning Mocktail recipe and home acupressure point (found in month two).
- You may want to start a pregnancy or dream journal.
- Consider joining a pregnancy forum or group, online or in-person.
- Start some financial planning for your family.

What Is the Placenta, Anyway?

The placenta is a link between you and baby. In some cultures, the placenta is referred to as "little mother." This organ, which embeds in your uterus and connects to the baby by the umbilical cord, works to support your baby throughout pregnancy. The placenta is responsible for the exchange of oxygen and nutrients between you and baby's blood and develops from some of the same cells that are in your uterine walls, as well as cells from the developing baby. So it really is a mixture of you and baby. This little helper also produces hormones that help your baby grow and develop, and just like your baby, the placenta grows throughout pregnancy.

The first hormone produced by the placenta is human chorionic gonadotropin (hCG), which is what's being measured in a positive pregnancy test. hCG also ensures that the corpus luteum of the implanting embryo continues to secrete progesterone and estrogen to signal to the body not to have a period (progesterone is produced by the placenta for this reason as well). Other wonders of hCG are that it suppresses your autoimmune response so that your body doesn't reject the placenta or baby. The placenta also produces human placental lactogen (hPL) and estrogen, which both contribute to the development of your mammary glands in early preparation for lactation.

The placenta provides some immune protection for baby against most bacteria, but not viruses. That's why contracting a virus such as chicken pox can be very dangerous during pregnancy. The passive immunity you pass on to baby lingers for a few months after birth, which is why the health of your immune system is an imperative piece of baby's immune system.

Other things that can adversely affect baby via the placenta are obesity and gestational diabetes, which can increase or decrease levels of nutrients transported to the baby and result in overgrowth or restricted growth of baby. Alcohol, nicotine, and other drugs can cross the placental barrier and cause damage to the baby. If they're in your life, it's time to give them up.

During birth, the placenta separates from the wall of the uterus and is birthed after your baby. This usually occurs about fifteen to thirty minutes after baby's birth. Letting baby suckle right away (most babies can find their way on their own to the nipple if given ample opportunity on the chest after birth) can help stimulate contractions that help pass the placenta. Many women opt to keep the baby on their chest during this time, with the umbilical cord still attached to the placenta, to allow all of the nutrients to pass through. What's passing through is also known as cord blood, which is sometimes harvested and banked. Unless personal choices or family history warrant saving your cord blood, there is no medical reason to cut the cord immediately after birth, and not cutting it may help the baby's immune system adapt to life outside the uterus.

Some stuff that can go awry with the placenta:

- Placenta accrete: when the placenta implants too deeply into the uterine wall

- Placenta praevia: when the placenta is too close to or blocking the cervix

- Placental abruption: when the placenta separates from the lining of the uterus before it's supposed to

- Placentitis: includes various infections that can pass to baby

A note on the umbilical cord: Normally this conduit between the baby and the placenta contains two arteries and one vein for supplying oxygen and sustenance to the baby, but occasionally there can be a single umbilical artery. If this happens, you will most likely want to seek out a fetal echocardiogram to monitor the baby's heart, since the oxygen flow is reduced and this presentation can sometimes increase the risk of congenital heart disease (CHD) in baby.

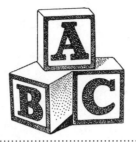

Month Two
Processing

WEEK NINE

- Baby is .9 inches and .07 ounces.
- Brain waves can be detected by an electroencephalogram (EEG).
- The skeleton is formed.
- Fingers and toes are fully defined.

WEEK TEN

- Baby is 1.2 inches and .14 ounces.
- Almost all organs are completely formed, and kidneys begin to function.
- The fetus can move and respond to touch when prodded through your abdomen.
- Arm joints are functioning.
- Hair and fingernails are growing.
- Baby is already practicing swallowing.

WEEK ELEVEN

- Baby is 1.6 inches and .25 ounces.
- The head and body are proportional (for now).
- Fingers and toes are no longer webbed.

....

WEEK TWELVE

- Baby is 2.1 inches and .49 ounces.
- Reflexes are continuing to develop.
- Fingers and toes are wiggling.

....

East-West Fetal Development

This month of the baby's development correlates to the Chinese Gallbladder system, which carries with it the emotional themes of change, processing, and decision making. You may have noticed yourself having different reactions to change than you're used to, or more than usual moodiness. Don't fret. You're working overtime, and expressing a full range of whatever emotions may be present for you is an important part of ultimately more smoothly processing these physical and emotional changes. You're not harming your baby by being in an unpredictable mood.

Just as you are working overtime, your actual gallbladder is clocking a lot of time as well. It may have difficulty processing greasy, fatty foods. You might find yourself beginning to veer toward a vegetarian diet, no matter how much of a carnivore you used to be. Just get protein where you can (remember quinoa is a protein too!). The upcoming chapters will be chock-full of recipes with vegetarian slants to help you get adequate pregnancy nutrition without disrespecting your aversions.

It may be hard to see the forest for the trees right now (especially because visual changes can occur during this month), but while you're surviving these rigors, some pivotal decisions need to be made about how to proceed with genetic testing and how to manage a general life balance that's conducive to the rest and support you need to finish your first trimester.

Now that you've had a little time to adjust to being pregnant, it might be time to adjust some of your patterns and shift into new routines that make room for all that is required of you and your body right now. This may include relaxing into the back-and-forth flux while incorporating new ways of thinking, eating, or even feeling.

Did You Know Your Partner May Be Going Through Pregnancy Too?

Couvade, a derivative of the Breton verb *couver*—to brood or incubate—is a legitimate syndrome in which your significant other, whose empathy you may usually appreciate, complains of the same or similar symptoms to you. Of course, he doesn't have the actual pregnancy excuse, so it might be hard to fully sympathize with him in the throes (or throwing up) of your own experience.

Prodding aside, there are references dating back to 60 BCE of fathers being prescribed bed rest because they had signs mimicking labor—the most common consensus of symptoms with today's modern father being weight gain, cravings, flatulence, and toothaches.

So, be gentle with each other, as you're both adjusting to this major life change, which can trigger all sorts of reactions. And kudos for the men of couvade—they're as participatory as it comes.

Ultrasounds

Although regular checkups are recommended during pregnancy, that doesn't necessarily mean regular ultrasounds at each checkup. Ultrasounds can provide important information and even allow you to begin to bond to baby. It can be exciting to gather this first bit of evidence, and, it's important to evaluate the benefits and risks of this keepsake scan.

Ultrasounds have been used in obstetrics for a few decades without major evidence of harm. We often hear mixed input about the potential harm ultrasounds may be doing, and an absence of evidence of harm is not the same thing as *evidence of absence of harm*. In this case though, there really only is a smattering of research around a high frequency of ultrasounds potentially contributing to low birth weight (and it is worth noting that many factors may contribute to low birth weight). Also, it can be hard to isolate one cause of low birth weight, and more importantly, babies can rapidly recover from this. Oddly, the only other consistent finding with ultrasounds in utero is that boys exposed to frequent ultrasounds are more likely to be left-handed (obviously not a medical problem).

You may have also heard the myth that when a baby hears an ultrasound, it sounds as loud as a subway train. In truth, the pulsing from ultrasounds would probably translate, to baby, as a pitch and rhythm that's similar to tapping the highest notes on a piano. Ultrasounds do produce heat and pressure changes in there. Your baby is kind of like a deep-sea diver, and the negative pressure of ultrasounds can produce gas bubbles equivalent to a diver's decompression. In very, very rare instances, this can lead to tissue damage at the site of the bubble. These impacts are most relevant to a developing embryo (preimplantation) and in later stages of pregnancy when the baby has more mineralization in her bones, which can absorb more of the radiation exposure.

For this reason, you may want to consider not having an ultrasound too early, and minimize the late pregnancy ultrasounds unless a known medical condition warrants it. Even though it's exciting to see your baby splashing around, now that you know that his intriguing movement during the ultrasound might be a response to the invasion of his quiet space, perhaps it will temper your temptation to see what your child is doing at every given moment. However, to introduce one of many conflicting stands, as the nature of pregnancy is to work in the gray areas, sometimes assuaging your own worry is actually worth some minor intervention, and having said all of this, I'd like to reiterate that the current risk of ultrasounds is incredibly low, and technology is constantly being improved and refined. So, don't be dissuaded from getting any necessary diagnostics.

Intrauterine Growth Restriction (IUGR)

When the baby isn't growing as expected it can be a very scary feeling, and the truth is, it can represent significant and life-threatening problems for the baby. Carefully monitoring the baby and assessing factors such as her blood flow supply and overall well-being will be the cornerstone of differentiating temporary growth changes that aren't exactly on the curve versus true IUGR.

Did You Know You Can Measure Your Baby's Growth at Home?

It is often comforting to get some regular, tangible information to support your developing trust in your pregnancy. Uterine growth is correlated to the growth of your baby, and you can measure this at home. Use a soft tape measure to measure the distance from your pubic bone to the top of your uterus, or *fundus*. You can usually feel the fundus if you start at the midline of your stomach, by your belly button, then gently push inward as you move your hand down, until it feels like you push against something. The number in centimeters from the top of your pubic bone to the top of your uterus should correlate pretty closely to the number of weeks of your pregnancy.

So, if you're twenty weeks along (about to the belly button), you will measure at about 20 centimeters. Don't worry if there's a little give or take. This is not a precise science, and in-utero babies, just like children, grow at different rates and paces within the normal range. Any measurements outside of 2 centimeters, or two weeks off, should be brought to the attention of your care provider for further discussion. Don't leap to any conclusions based on one measurement.

Nausea and Vomiting

Colloquially known as "morning sickness" despite being an omnipresent daily event for many expecting women, nausea (which sometimes, but not always, includes vomiting) affects 90 percent of pregnant women at some point in their pregnancy, and its impact is often sorely underappreciated in regard to the misery and disruption of daily life. "Morning sickness" is a complete misnomer; it can strike at any time. It's crucial to remember that you're not sick—you're pregnant and healthy; you just have nausea and vomiting.

On that note, perhaps the experience of nausea and vomiting is more adaptive than it is pathological. The earliest descriptions of vomiting during pregnancy date from about 2,000 BCE, which gives us a clue as to the origins of this curious effect of pregnancy. As with many anthropological explanations, a biological rationale exists. Nausea, vomiting, and the heightened sense of smell that are often present in the early stages of pregnancy have all been postulated to be protective mechanisms to prevent women from consuming substances that could be harmful to the fetus.

For example, many newly pregnant women feel repulsed by the thought of eating animal products. There is a logical reason for this: meat and dairy, traditionally, often contained pathogens and parasites that could harm the developing fetus. Of course, in our modern world, this is unlikely, but remember that your body is reacting based on its genetic legacy. A few hundred years ago—before the advent of refrigerators and modern food sanitation techniques—animal products stored at room temperature could be dangerous for pregnant women to consume. Even though food poisoning might blend right in with nausea and vomiting, let's not add insult to injury.

An aversion to animal-based food products is, of course, only one potential scenario, and many women experience quite the opposite effect. Morning sickness, cravings, and aversions are seemingly random and unique to each pregnant woman, but it can be comforting to know that they are happening for a very good reason—albeit one that may be a relic of our anthropological development.

Indeed, symptoms of nausea and vomiting often seem to peak when babies are most susceptible to harmful changes from chemical disruption (weeks six to eighteen). A pregnant woman's immune response is weakened during pregnancy in order to prevent her body from rejecting its own offspring. A fetus contains half of another genetic body's immune system, so the carrying mother's body can see it as a foreign organism. This immune susceptibility is also why pregnant women (and their babies) are at greater risk for food-borne pathogens such as toxoplasmosis.

As pregnancy progresses, you'll probably notice that your food aversions decrease, paralleling the strengthening of your and your child's immunity. Another explanation for random food aversions may be that your body is acting on behalf of potential allergies in your fetus. Yet, another theory is that nausea corresponds to rising levels of the pregnancy hormone human chorionic gonadotropin (hCG).

The silver lining in the stomach lining: except for an unlucky 10 percent of women whose symptoms last right up to birth, is that most women do spontaneously improve and don't have any long-term consequences to

Acupressure Relief

There is a traditional acupressure point that can help relieve nausea. You can find this on yourself by bending your index finger and placing the bend of your knuckle on the inside of your wrist, right in the middle of your wrist crease. Where the tip of your finger (not nail) falls, in-between the two main tendons (you may have to make a fist to make them more visible) is the acupressure point known as *Nei Guan* or "Inner Pass," which I interpret in this context as giving you a pass on nausea. Press your thumb firmly into this point or have someone else apply pressure for you. (It will probably be sensitive.) Retain this pressure for at least a few minutes and stimulate as needed throughout your day. If you're opting for trying out a nausea wristband, make sure the nub falls on this location as well.

Acupuncture often helps both the physical symptoms and potential emotional distress of nausea, and psychotherapy and hypnotherapy can provide relief from the psychological rigor that can erode your stamina during this time. For many women in my practice, yoga, walking, or other movement helps with morning sickness. But for some women, unfortunately, nothing seems to help. The good news? It gets better (most of the time)! Just hang in there.

their pregnancy as a result of morning sickness. Many of my patients have reported to me that they woke up one day (usually on the cusp of the second trimester) and their morning sickness was magically and permanently gone. This will probably happen for you too.

In the meantime, mild to medium cases of nausea can generally be managed by eating enough protein and staying hydrated. Of course, while both of these things can help stave off nausea to whatever extent is available, often the last thing one wants during this time is protein, which leads to what I call the "beige diet" (more on that below). For now, your mantra should simply be "this too shall pass," and your M.O. to eat what you want and can stomach—as long as it includes a prenatal vitamin that contains folic acid, which can adequately support an important aspect of baby's development during this time of monotonous food intake.

Severe Nausea and Vomiting

Up to 2 percent of pregnant women experience persistent and intense nausea and vomiting, known in medical circles as *hyperemesis gravidarum*. Some women at this stage might even be so disconsolate that they feel a desire to terminate their pregnancy. That's how unmanageable so-called "morning sickness" can be.

Signs of severity include nausea and vomiting that continue beyond the first trimester or simply feel unmanageable to you. If severe, the situation demands intervention. You could lose a significant amount of electrolytes, which will threaten you and baby's nutritional needs. This could call for intravenous fluids for electrolyte replacement, vitamin B1 supplementation, potential use of conventional antinausea medication (antiemetics), and psychological support to develop strategies for dealing with the discomfort and learning to navigate it—because let's face it, inability to comfortably function in your daily life is bound to make any woman feel unstable.

It's important to involve the right interventions of skilled clinicians for management, encouragement, and support.

Diet for Morning Sickness

In Chinese medicine, we advocate a balanced diet—which includes good quality meat—for most pregnant women. But many women, at this point, involuntarily convert to what I call the "beige diet," with a focus on crackers, bread, rice, etc. You might normally have a varied diet with a love of vegetables and balanced nutrition, but don't be surprised if your body starts to reject the things you once thought were delicious once you are pregnant. Since food is such a comfort for us, and we all have our attachments to foods that we believe make us feel better, this can add another confounding layer. Take comfort in knowing that many cravings are related to actual nutritional needs; harken back to chocolate cravings during PMS (chocolate contributes magnesium, which is great for relaxing cramping), and carbohydrates (the "beige foods") trigger the release of insulin, which promotes the absorption of amino acids, such as tryptophan (also contained in eggs, salmon, nuts, and seeds), which gives you a serotonin boost and makes you feel good, which goes a long way in pregnancy. These foods become relevant again toward the end of pregnancy when they may help prepare for birth on the backdrop of very little room in your stomach.

Many women express concern during this time that they are not giving their baby the nutrients it needs. If you're trying your best to get the foundations from the "eat like you're taking a prenatal vitamin" section of this book, you're in good shape. Like a picky toddler who sometimes refuses the wholesome food choices given to him, you will survive, and you will, in fact, be fine—and so will your baby—as long as you get some of the basic building blocks down the hatch. As your appetite restores itself, typically in the second trimester, you will make up for all of this "bad eating."

However, note that during this early stage of pregnancy, eating protein and staying really hydrated can, for many women, stave off nausea and vomiting to some degree. Even though small, protein-based meals—if you can manage them—will often quell a certain degree of nausea, the difficult irony during this time is that, once nausea sets in, the last thing most women crave is protein, and sometimes even things as innocuous as water seem repulsive. So, again, the first trimester is a good time to practice letting go. There's really nothing for you to do but sink into the changes happening to your body, rest as much as you can get away with, and nourish yourself as best you can.

For those of you not able to stomach the thought of eating meat, here's a consolation bit of research for you: morning sickness has never been observed in societies with a primary dietary staple of only plants (mainly, corn). Let's not go crazy about corn though. Besides being hard to digest, if it's spoiled, it can produce microorganisms that are harmful to fetuses. Think of the corn factor more as a metaphor for the permission to eat bland veggies and grains. So, if any of the things that are supposedly "good for you" sound absolutely intolerable in your given state of queasiness, rest assured that you will have time to play catch-up with nutrition in your next trimester. In the meantime, I've included in this chapter a recipe for porridge that can be a medium for toppings that can impart some good and palatable nutrition right now.

Lethargy and Sluggishness

We've talked about sluggishness in your body, but this myopic view doesn't account for the *whole you* feeling lethargic. From the start, I'd like to remind you that you are actually growing a whole person, and this takes a huge amount of your resources. It can be challenging to remember this, since your pregnancy may still seem like an abstract concept, but let me assure you, it's happening, and it's requiring almost all of you.

This is an important time to begin to adjust your relationship to what you're able to do—which does not mean you're in any way incompetent. The most active, busy women find themselves yearning to be sedentary during this time. You will inevitably have energy shifts throughout your pregnancy, allowing you more of a semblance of the *you* that you knew yourself to be. But the first trimester is a time to slow down, at least a bit, and let your body do what it needs to do. There's no cure (because it's not an ailment; it's just a healthy albeit uncomfortable process), not even sleep. You can push through, but you can also choose to revel to some degree in this inevitable part of your pregnancy by finding ways to indulge in this new pace in any way you can. I promise the world, and all that you may be doing in the world, will go on. This is a pause, but not a permanent stop. This particular quality of fatigue will most likely begin to lift in the second trimester.

Slowing down brings up a lot for most people. Most of us define ourselves in some manner by what we do or how we do things. This is a wonderful time to connect with the inherent value inside yourself that is not just attached to what you do.

Ptyalism (Drooling)

Unique disorders are associated with pregnancy. One of these is ptyalism, less delicately known as drooling. During the first trimester, when the whole digestive tract is in upheaval, this can be an uncouth side effect.

One possible culprit of ptyalism is the sympathetic nervous system, which is responsible for our fight-or-flight reaction to stress. Unfortunately, there's no running away from this symptom, which some women experience as an embarrassing but really rather harmless side effect of pregnancy. In addition to your nerves being shot, nausea and heartburn can stimulate the salivary glands to produce excess saliva in an attempt to protect the throat and mouth from the irritation of acid reflux and vomiting. If you've been forced to resort to carrying around a spittoon, at least the acid in your stomach may have neutralized.

....

ANCIENT GRAIN PORRIDGE

Ingredients

> 1 cup mixture of grains such as buckwheat, barley, farro, quinoa, millet and amaranth
>
> 3 cups water
>
> ¼ teaspoon salt
>
> ¾ cup dried berries (blueberries, cherries, etc.)
>
> 2 cinnamon sticks
>
> 1 vanilla bean (or ¼ teaspoon real vanilla extract)

Directions

Rinse the grains in hot water. Bring water and salt to a boil. Add grains and the rest of the ingredients to the water, turn down to low heat, and cook covered for fifteen minutes. Stir occasionally. When the water is gone, cover and turn off the heat. The porridge should be just about ready in another ten minutes. Remove the cinnamon sticks and vanilla bean, and mix in almond milk or coconut milk. (You can reuse the spices the next morning if you rinse them in cold water and let them dry.)

Nutritious topping ideas: Chia, flax, or pumpkin seeds; shredded coconut; walnuts; a tablespoon of blackstrap molasses; seasonal fruit.

....

As you may recall from month one, the Chinese Liver system is analogous to the nervous system. So, nourishing yourself with activities such as walking, yoga, or anything that helps keep stress coursing through your body may diminish the production of salvia. Chewing gum sometimes helps as well, and the only other advice I can give you for drooling is to optimize your digestion and do your best to manage other symptoms such as nausea and reflux to whatever extent possible.

NOTE: Antacids such as Tums and Mylanta, famotidine (Pepcid), and andranitidine (Zantac) are generally thought to be safe to use during pregnancy, but always consult with your doctor before using any medication and bear in mind these are palliative, not curative remedies. Over time they can actually alter your stomach acid and worsen the problem, which is why many of the recipes in this book are aimed at strengthening your digestion.

Keeping an Eye on Pregnancy

You may feel like you're flying blind right now, and another in the slew of unexpected symptoms can be changes in your vision. All of the same changes that are essential for supporting the baby can also contribute to a spectrum of not-so-favorable changes for you—especially on the visual spectrum.

Fluid retention during pregnancy can actually change the thickness and shape of your cornea, contributing to a little distortion in your vision. In Chinese medicine, we say that the Liver opens to the eyes, and you may recall that the first trimester kicks off the Liver's action, which weaves into this month as well, since the Liver is a kindred pairing to the Gallbladder.

The Chinese Liver system also supplies blood flow to the uterus (read: blood flow rerouted from everywhere else). In Chinese medicine, this idea of blood flow also encompasses other fluids, such as the ones that lubricate your eyes, and one of the primary visual problems that can occur right now (which typically self-resolves after pregnancy) is the development of dry eyes and blurry vision.

As a matter of fact, in Chinese medicine we call dry eyes "Liver blood deficiency." Breast milk is also related to this fluid level. So, boosting up and nourishing now can help you way down the line as well.

To nourish this "blood" level, foods from the iron-rich category in month one can boost you up and help you see straight. You can also use "artificial tears" to lubricate your eyes. Just make sure to check with your doctor to make sure the active ingredients are safe for you.

Other ocular (eye) issue that can happen during pregnancy can be thought of in three categories:

1. Visual changes that occur for the first time during pregnancy, such as increased pigmentation around the eye.

2. Existing issues that are further exacerbated or changed by pregnancy—such as diabetes, which can lead to diabetic retinopathy during pregnancy.

Recipes for Eye Relief

A good old-fashioned cucumber soak can be a soothing topical relief for agitated eyes. You can also make tea from an herb aptly named *eyebright*. Place a handful of the bulk herb in a pot of water and let simmer for about fifteen minutes. Strain through muslin cloth and—important!—make sure there aren't any particles left. Cool this concoction in the fridge and use as an eyewash one to two times per day by decanting some of the strained tea into another vessel and either splashing it generously on your eyes or by soaking a clean cloth and letting it rest over your eyes.

3. Visual changes that can be clues about other conditions, such as pre-eclampsia (this condition can damage the small blood vessels that supply the retinas of the eyes, causing a particular strain of visual changes such as temporary loss of vision, persistent light sensitivity, auras, or the appearance of flashing lights).

4. Eclampsia, Sheehan syndrome, or Grave's disease.

One positive effect that pregnancy can have on the eyes: if you suffer from an immune-related condition that affects the eyes, pregnancy can be a period of reprieve, since it's generally a time of relative immune suppression.

Check in with your provider about any visual changes but don't count on getting your prescription changed or of course plan any eye surgeries during pregnancy. Wait a few months after birth, because most of these issues will self-resolve. In the meantime, wearing sunglasses and minimizing screen time can bring some relief to overstrained eyes. You can also drink plenty of carrot, spinach, and kale juice—a great blend of lutein-rich foods that contribute health and vitality to your eyes.

Nervousness about Genetic Testing

Genetic testing is a very personal choice for you and your partner. In addition to considerations such as age, ethnic background, and health history, all of which influence potential genetic concerns for your baby, these decisions are also intertwined with your emotions and your personal values. Being faced with genetic testing can be one of your first steps in developing an emotional lexicon around parenting. It's great prep for what you will have to deal with from here on out: never getting a right or wrong answer from "experts," but instead having to always arrive at the answer that's right for your family, through weighing the options. It's also great preparation for the stress that you will come to know as a normal part of parenting.

Science has made it possible for us to find out a lot about a baby long before it is born. However, it's important to remember that science isn't perfect and there is still a lot we do not know. And needing to know the answers at a time when it is not always possible to get them is a direct recipe for suffering. This is why, in this chapter, we will start to emphasize the option of not only relying on scientific information but also touching in on your own truths as you make decisions about your pregnancy and which tests to conduct.

On the very slim chance that genetic testing causes you to encounter a potential abnormality in your baby, the type of decision making you will be faced with will be complex and emotional. So, I recommend seeking out a therapist who specializes in these issues to help you navigate the gray areas, and remember that you're always in charge of what's right for you.

There are many layers to both the testing and the decision making process. In an attempt to help you weigh the benefits and risks, here are some of the statistics and reasons for the typical interventions that you have to choose from for your screenings, and also some help interpreting the statistics. A genetic counselor can also be a great resource to help you weed through all of the statistics and variables.

Tips and a Guided Exercise for Approaching the Questions of Genetic Testing

The process of approaching whether or not to do none, all, or some of the available tests for helping determine the likely genetic outcome of your child is a question-and-answer process that is unique for everyone. There is no right answer, only what is right for you. So, to help guide you toward knowing more about what is right for you, here are some questions designed to give you the freedom to explore the possibilities. I also recommend, if applicable, sharing this exercise with your partner so that you can compare notes and arrive at a decision that is mutual and involves both of your beliefs, hopes, and desires.

Take at least ten minutes for each question and write about whatever comes up for you when posed with each question.

1. Are you comfortable with relatively noninvasive/low-risk initial testing (blood tests such as MaterniT21 and ultrasound) to gain a starting place for determining how to proceed with further genetic testing?

2. Based on the information above, if you got borderline/inconclusive information back, would you desire more conclusive information even if it carried a small risk to the pregnancy itself (amniocentesis or chorionic villus sampling)?

3. If you found out your baby had a genetic abnormality, would you consider terminating this pregnancy?

4. If considering retaining your pregnancy in the face of an abnormal finding, do you feel that some genetic abnormalities are more tolerable than others?

5. Are there any circumstances under which you would absolutely not terminate?

6. Are there circumstances under which you would absolutely terminate?

7. How do your feelings or instincts about your pregnancy match up to what you think you *should* do?

8. If there are any discrepancies in the above questions, are there any bridges between these different feelings and thoughts?

Take a few minutes to reflect on your answers, and perhaps share with your partner—knowing that this is the foundation of a conversation that may change in the upcoming weeks as you near the time to make each of these choices. Set aside a time for yourself once a week to review these questions, alone or together, and see if anything changes for you. Allow yourself and each other to be the guides for the parenting that is right for your unique family.

There are typical times associated with screening different aspects of your pregnancy, as follows:

First Trimester Tests

In the first trimester, most people are anxious to get some markers for how their pregnancy is going. It is often tempting to satiate our anxieties with information, but nothing in this process of genetic testing is black and white—except, of course, the ultrasound photograph. However, outside of our own relationship to reassurance, since there are few other things to go on, screening can be a very comforting process, and if you have a partner, it can be a way for both of you to have a tangible glimpse of the growing baby and potentially connect more closely to what's happening inside your body.

We've all heard the adage that women become mothers the moment they find out they're pregnant, and that men or partners become parents when they're holding their baby. I have noticed in my own practice with countless couples that many partners experience a more relatable connection to the pregnancy when they see the first ultrasound. "There's a baby in there!" At which point, you look at them as if to say, that's what I've been telling you for weeks. So, this test can be a relatively tangible way for each of you to begin to gain a relationship and trust in the health of your developing baby. Remember, each test is one piece of the pie, and a comprehensive set of information over time is what will best inform you. So, if there is an initially unfavorable result in one area, hang in there while you gather more evidence (and of course always retest negative results as lab errors can occur as well).

The least invasive, first set of tests is an integrated screening combining an ultrasound and blood tests. When used together, the tests (below) can help to both confirm a healthy pregnancy and begin to identify potential risks of certain birth defects such as Down syndrome (trisomy 21), Edwards syndrome (trisomy 18), and Patau syndrome (trisomy 13).

HUMAN CHORIONIC GONADOTROPIN HORMONE (HCG)

hCG is not only an indicator of pregnancy, but also a hormone produced by the placenta. An unexpected number can simply suggest a miscalculated due date, but a high level can also indicate the possibility of multiples or, in rare cases, a molar pregnancy. A very low level may indicate the threat of a miscarriage, or an ectopic pregnancy.

OTHER BLOOD TESTS

One standard blood test measures substances found in all pregnant women during early pregnancy. Abnormal levels are associated with an increased risk in chromosomal abnormalities.

- Pregnancy-associated plasma protein screening (PAPP-A)

There are also specialized blood tests, which have higher detection rates and lower false-positive rates than other first trimester screenings.

- MaterniT21, Harmony, Verifi, and Panorama all measure fetal chromosomal abnormalities and can also detect the sex of the baby as early as ten weeks in.

NUCHAL TRANSLUCENCY (NT)

This is a topical ultrasound that looks at the back of your baby's neck to rule out any skin thickness and increased fluid accumulation. If the nuchal translucency is in the 95th percentile or measures more than 3.5 mm, it is considered an increased risk factor for chromosomal abnormalities, congenital heart malformations, Noonan syndrome, and, ultimately, pregnancy loss.

Keep in mind that very occasionally there can be "false positive" results, indicating a problem when the fetus is actually healthy, and there can also be "false negative" results, indicating no abnormality when the fetus actually does have a health problem. If the outcome of the tests won't affect your decision about keeping your pregnancy, then there may be less reason to have further tests such as chorionic villus sampling or amniocentesis. Although, knowing about any potential risk, even if it doesn't change your decision to have the baby, may help you with additional preparations. However, if any of the above results are abnormal, and that might influence your decision about your pregnancy, then some of your complex decision making about the next levels of screening may commence. In addition to using our guided exercise for coming up with your own insights, you may also want to seek out genetic counseling and any other support that helps you to further inform your choices.

Second Trimester Tests

From weeks fifteen to twenty-two, you can have several optional blood tests (most accurate when done between weeks sixteen to eighteen), called the

Do You Know Why You Have to Pee in a Cup at Almost Every Prenatal Visit?

Here's what's being tested at different stages of pregnancy through your urine, and why:

• Red blood cells: to look for urinary tract disease

• White blood cells: to look for urinary tract infection

• Glucose: to look for sugar imbalance or diabetes

• Protein: to look for signs of preeclampsia

"multiple marker screening," which continues to provide information about potential genetic conditions or birth defects such as Down syndrome, trisomy 18, and neural tube defects.

All of the following tests together are called the quadruple screening.

ALPHA-FETOPROTEIN SCREENING (AFP)

Alpha-fetoprotein (AFP) is a protein produced by the baby's liver and present in the amniotic fluid. It crosses the placental barrier and is present in the mother's blood, which is why it is also called maternal serum alpha-fetoprotein (MSAFP). Increased levels of AFP can be a first indicator of some of the following. I can't emphasize enough—if you get an unfavorable result back, further screening is necessary before leaping to any conclusions:

• Down syndrome and other chromosomal abnormalities

• A miscalculated due date or multiples

• Defect in the baby's intestines or other nearby organs

• Potential miscarriage

• Open neural tube defects (ONTD) and spinal defects such as spina bifida

• Tetralogy of Fallot (heart defect)

• Turner syndrome (genetic defect)

• Absence of part of the brain and skull (anencephaly)

ESTRIOL

This is a hormone produced by the placenta and your baby's liver. Significantly lower than normal levels of estriol may indicate an increased risk of Down syndrome.

INHIBIN-A

This is a hormone produced by the placenta. Low levels of AFP and estriol, along with high levels of hCG and inhibin-A, may be due to issues such as:

- Down syndrome (trisomy 21)

- Edwards syndrome (trisomy 18)

If this last test is omitted, then it's called a triple screening. The results of the triple/quadruple screening are usually given as a probability of risk. Generally, the test is considered positive if the risk is one in 300 or less. Multiple marker screening is not diagnostic. It is only a screening test to assist you in determining if you might want additional, more definitive testing and is integrated with your cumulative tests for a more comprehensive assessment.

Keep in mind that a positive test (meaning negative results) simply means that some of the levels that were measured were outside the normal range. Again, this is not definitive and can happen for many reasons, including:

- A miscalculation of how long you've been pregnant

- The presence of multiples

- Hormone changes in your blood from in vitro fertilization (IVF)

- The presence of other medical conditions, such as diabetes

MaterniT21 (and related tests in this category), amniocentesis, and chorionic villus sampling can help further diagnose genetic disorders such as cystic fibrosis, Down syndrome, muscular dystrophy, sickle cell anemia, Tay-Sachs disease, neural tube defects, hemophilia A, and thalassemia.

CHORIONIC VILLUS SAMPLING (CVS) AND AMNIOCENTESIS

Chorionic villus sampling (CVS) extracts a sample of placental tissue, which contains the same genetic material as the baby and can be tested for chromosomal abnormalities and genetic disorders. It is either done with a catheter through the vagina and into the cervix to reach the uterus, or similarly to an amniocentesis, by needle insertion through the abdomen into the uterus.

This procedure is usually done between weeks ten and twelve because earlier testing has been linked to some reports of causing limb abnormalities in the baby.

Sometimes a CVS sample doesn't yield enough tissue to examine in the laboratory, so the results can be inconclusive and may warrant an amniocentesis as well. Additionally, if you have an active vaginal infection such as herpes or gonorrhea, it is prohibitive for having a CVS. In comparison to amniocentesis, CVS does not provide information on neural tube defects such as spina bifida. The second trimester blood tests listed above will continue to screen for neural tube defects.

If you opt for an amniocentesis, it is usually performed between weeks fifteen and twenty. This involves a needle biopsy through your abdomen into the amniotic sac to gather a sample of the amniotic fluid, which contains cells that have been shed by the baby and alpha-fetoprotein (a protein made by the baby). Through this method, more reliable genetic detection of chromosomal disorders and open neural tube defects (ONTDs) such as spina bifida can be obtained.

If you are carrying multiples, you can expect multiple samples to be needed from each placenta or amniotic sac, but this isn't always possible due to positioning of the babies, location of the placenta, amount of amniotic fluid, or your own anatomy.

The main risks (albeit small) that CVS and amniocentesis carry are increased risks for pregnancy loss and possible risks for birth defects. On average, pregnancy loss after a CVS is 1.1 percent (about one out of every 100 women) and amniocentesis 0.4 percent (about one out of every 1,400 women). The risks are low, but they do exist. After all of the above procedures, strenuous activities should be avoided for at least twenty-four hours. Typically, you'll get your results back in about ten days.

Waiting for results can be an anxiety-inducing process, but it can also be an opportunity to cultivate your relationship to the decisions you face independent of being influenced by the results at this stage. This is a great time to utilize the genetic testing writing exercise found earlier in this chapter and any other tools that you find helpful for arriving at a clear choice, or at least an avenue toward peace of mind for yourself.

A Note on Genetic Testing if You've Gone through In-Vitro Fertilization (IVF)

If you've done preimplantation genetic diagnosis (PGD) or comprehensive chromosome screening (CCS) during IVF, it certainly minimizes your risks of having a baby with abnormal chromosomes, but it is still advisable to go through the basic pregnancy screening processes if that is in alignment with the overall route of pregnancy screening that you're choosing.

FETAL BLOOD SAMPLING (FBS)

FBS is the collection of blood directly from the umbilical cord, which is tested for signs that your immune system is attacking the baby's red blood cells (which is only possible, by the way, if you are Rh-sensitized and your baby is Rh-positive). A slight risk of this procedure is that it can lead to worsening of the Rh-sensitization problems, since the baby's blood may mix with the mother's blood during the blood sampling, and you may need to take medications to help prevent preterm labor (tocolytic medicines) for this procedure.

Gestational Diabetes

Normal metabolic changes occur throughout pregnancy, mostly to help optimize the transfer of nutrients to the baby. One of them is a decrease in insulin sensitivity, which requires an increase in insulin production to counteract this change and keep glucose (blood sugar) balanced for mom and baby. When this balance doesn't occur and glucose is too high, the result can be gestational diabetes mellitus (GDM). GDM is the most common medical complication of pregnancy.

Some of the hormones involved in this process include estrogen, progesterone, cortisol, and prolactin, which increase and promote pancreatic changes and insulin release, resulting in higher fasting glucose, or higher blood sugar levels. Each of these hormones has a peak time that it affects the glucose balance. For instance, cortisol peaks in its effect at twenty-six weeks of gestation, and progesterone has strong anti-insulin properties that peak at thirty-two weeks. The timing of these hormonal changes is relevant in scheduling your testing for GDM.

Diagnosing and treating GDM is important for preventing any adverse outcomes, such as:

- Polyhydramnios (excessive accumulation of amniotic fluid)
- Macrosomia (abnormally large growth of the baby)
- Early delivery
- Increased risk of cesarean section, because the particular growth pattern that occurs from glucose imbalances can create a larger shoulder girth compared to head circumference in babies and contribute to an increase in the risk of shoulder dystocia during birth

As a side note, studies have shown that there is a correlation between rates of shoulder dystocia and birth weight. If the estimated weight of your baby is over 9.9 pounds, it may play an important role in the decision-making process for route of delivery. But just remember that ultrasounds have a range of error of about 10 to 15 percent in estimating fetal weight at term.

So, although GDM can set you and your baby up for postpartum blood-sugar issues, continued monitoring throughout your pregnancy and after birth (including a glucose-tolerance test six weeks after birth and a fasting glucose test annually) it usually results in very manageable and recoverable outcomes. Also, rest assured that GDM can be a normal course of development even with the healthiest of habits, so if you do test positive for it, it's not necessarily something you're doing or not doing.

Typical screening for GDM is performed with a 50 gram oral glucose load given between twenty-four and twenty-eight weeks. Basically, this is an artificially colored, very sweet drink that you have to manage to get down in about five minutes, followed by a blood draw an hour later to measure glucose levels in your blood. If your glucose is too high (over 140 mg/dl), you'll get further screening: a three-hour, 100-gram oral glucose tolerance test (OGTT). Women with high-risk factors, such as a prior personal or family history of diabetes or chronic steroid use, may benefit from earlier testing at around twenty weeks.

It is possible to get a false reading on your glucose test. So, if you have a high glucose level at one of your checkups, it's always a good idea to retest. Any of the factors below might contribute to a false reading:

- If you recently ate a larger meal than usual (especially carbohydrates such as bread, pasta, or rice) and haven't moved around much since eating
- If you ate within two hours of the test
- A contaminated urine sample
- If you already take insulin and missed a dose of your medication

As with many things, GDM can usually be successfully managed with a nutrition plan that emphasizes foods that are low on the glycemic index (GI). Carbohydrates are broken down at different rates. The glycemic index is a tool to understand and interpret how carbohydrates affect blood glucose levels (BGLs). For instance, foods that are high on the GI are broken down quickly and cause rapid rises in BGLs. Foods on the medium spectrum cause a moderate rise in BGLs, and foods low on the GI are just that— broken down slowly so that they create a small rise in BGLs, which is what you want for preventing or managing GDM. Additionally, consuming ten grams a day of fiber has been associated with a 26 percent reduction in the risk of GDM.

Eating well is key, since caloric restriction (a typical strategy for glycemic control) in pregnancy can increase ketone levels, which occur from the breakdown of fat instead of glucose, and can have negative effects on the baby. Other nutrients that are associated with preventing GDM include selenium, vitamin D, zinc, and myoinositol. The best sources for food-based myoinositol are beans, cantaloupe, citrus fruits (except lemons), grains, and nuts. For more variety, other foods that are particularly low on the glycemic index and good for managing blood sugar are:

asparagus	avocados
bamboo shoots	beef
blueberries	celery
cabbage	chicken

chlorophyll	daikon radishes
grapefruit	limes
shitake mushrooms	pears
plums	pumpkin
winter squash	radishes
snow peas	spinach
string beans	sweet potatoes
rice	millet
mung beans	toasted pumpkin seeds
turnips	

....

BALANCED MORNING PORRIDGE

Here's a Chinese porridge, or *jook*, that you can use as a base recipe to stabilize your blood sugar each morning, then add in whatever else appeals to you (preferably drawing on the list of foods low on the GI index). Jook, a bland and beige Chinese porridge, is a palatable way to get some digestible nutrients without aggravating an overstimulated stomach. It's very easy to make, for times when even standing up in the kitchen sounds challenging.

Ingredients

½ cup rice

½ cup quinoa (a grain that is also a complete protein)

8 cups water (you can also boost the nutrients by using the Boosted-Up Chicken Stock recipe on page 46 if you have some on hand and if it sounds yummy)

Three ¼-inch slices of fresh ginger root

Directions

Combine all ingredients in a large pot. Bring to a boil and let simmer for several hours or until the grains are well cooked. Use the back of a ladle or an immersion blender to mash the porridge into a soothing mush. Top with a poached egg (see next recipe).

....

....

POACHED EGGS

Fresh, pasture-raised eggs are the most nutrient-dense choice. If you can't find them, at least go for organic for maximum nutrition. A teaspoon of apple cider vinegar helps hold them together while you poach. In addition to topping your Balanced Morning Porridge, poached eggs can be eaten over steamed vegetables, with salads, with sprouted grain toast, or in soups.

Ingredients

Fresh pasture-raised or organic eggs

1 to 2 teaspoons apple cider vinegar

Pinch of sea salt

Equipment

Shallow saucepan with cover

Slotted spoon

Directions

Fill the saucepan with water and bring it to a boil. Then, lower the heat until the water is no longer boiling. Add vinegar to the water. Working with the eggs one by one, crack each egg into a small cup, then place the cup near the surface of the hot water and gently drop the egg into the water. With a spoon, nudge the egg whites closer to their yolks. This will continue to help the egg whites hold together. Turn off the heat. Cover. Let sit for four minutes, until the egg whites are cooked. Lift eggs out of pan with a slotted spoon.

....

Eating a balanced, protein-based breakfast paves the way for stable blood sugar throughout the day. Another pivotal strategy for managing GDM is to continue to eat protein-based meals, balanced with complex carbohydrate accompaniments that are low on the GI, and to get thirty minutes of physical activity every day, which helps to lower blood-glucose levels because your muscles are utilizing some of your circulating glucose.

QUINOA COOKIES

If you're feeling deprived while trying to manage your blood sugar, these cookies are a great, wholesome treat that still works in your favor.

Ingredients

  1 cup quinoa

  1 ½ cups water

  ½ banana

  1 heaping tablespoon roasted almond butter

  8 Medjool dates

  ¼ cup sunflower seeds

  ¼ cup pumpkin seeds

  ¼ cup shredded coconut

  3 sprinkles of cinnamon

  1 heaping tablespoon extra virgin coconut oil

Directions

Rinse quinoa, then combine with water in a medium pot. Bring to a boil, and then simmer for about twelve minutes. Preheat the oven to 350 degrees Fahrenheit. Transfer the quinoa to a large mixing bowl. Mix in coconut oil. Add chopped banana, almond butter, and dates, and mix. Add sunflower seeds, pumpkin seeds, and shredded coconut, and mix thoroughly. Sprinkle cinnamon into the dough and mix everything together. Grease a baking sheet with coconut oil.

Use a large spoon to pick up a heaping tablespoon of the dough and form it into a ball with your hands. Place the ball onto the greased cookie sheet and press the middle of the ball down gently to form a circle a bit more than a half inch thick. Repeat with the rest of the dough. Bake for fifty minutes. Remove cookies and allow to cool for fifteen minutes on baking sheet. You can store the cookies in an airtight container.

Snack Suggestion: Nut Butter

A good-quality nut butter such as almond, hazelnut, or sesame is a great way to get healthy fat and protein with your favorite fruits and vegetables. Try celery with almond butter, sprinkled with flax seeds.

Four grams per day of myoinositol plus 400 micrograms per day of folic acid taken for eight weeks has also been associated with significantly decreasing glucose levels. Low vitamin D levels have also been implicated. So check that too in case you need to add that into your supplement regime.

If attentive eating and exercise don't manage your GDM, sometimes insulin is indicated for treatment.

No Cons to Probiotics

From conception to long-term health, there is an ongoing interplay between genetics and environmental factors. During pregnancy, many of baby's immune functions are drawn from the mother's diet. Exchange of bacteria from the mother to the baby during pregnancy, birth, and breastfeeding influences baby's own intestinal flora, and a healthy start in this area may enhance baby's overall immunity and health later on. As a matter of fact, our highly hygienic conditions in the Western world, although they help prevent many diseases, can simultaneously be responsible for inhibiting proper maturation of the immune system and predispose a child to allergies and other immune susceptibilities.

Another pro for incorporating probiotics is that they may also interfere with the inflammatory cascade that can sometimes lead to preterm labor and delivery. Since there's no downside to utilizing probiotics throughout your pregnancy, I suggest either supplementing with a daily probiotic and/or regularly incorporating the following probiotic foods into your routine:

- Kefir (high in antioxidants, Bifidus bacteria, and Lactobacillus)
- Kimchi (a spicy and sour fermented cabbage with beneficial bacteria, high in beta-carotene, calcium, iron, and vitamins A, C, B1, and B2)

PROBIOTIC-RICH SOUP

A mainstay for easy probiotic consumption is miso soup. Miso is made from fermented rye, beans, rice, or barley. Simply adding it to hot water makes a quick, probiotic-rich soup full of Lactobacillus and bifidus bacteria.

Just scoop a heaping tablespoon of miso paste into some hot water (make sure it's cooled a little from the boiling point to preserve all the good effects of miso). For added nutrients, you can use your Boosted-Up Chicken Stock from month one as a base. As additions, you can stir in some sautéed or soaked (from dried) shitake mushrooms (these give you an extra immune boost) and sprinkle in some dried seaweed, such as dulse flakes.

Have a side of the following pickles for an extra probiotic boost with a refreshing crunch!

QUICK GINGER CARROT PICKLES

Ingredients

    10 carrots, cleaned but unpeeled

    4 inches of ginger, sliced lengthwise

    2 tablespoons sea salt

    3 cups of room-temperature water

Directions

Cut the carrots into quarters and put them in a quart-sized mason jar. Intersperse with slices of ginger in between the carrots. Dissolve salt into room-temperature water, and pour it over carrot and ginger pieces, filling up the jar so carrots and ginger are submerged. Try to leave about an inch of room between the surface of the liquid and the top of the jar. Cover with a fine mesh cloth and secure with a rubber band. Let sit at room temperature for one to two weeks, then use as a probiotic-rich side snack to accompany any of your other meals.

- Microalgae (ocean-based plants such as spirulina, chlorella, and blue-green algae, which are high in both Lactobacillus and Bifidus)

- Miso soup

- Pickles

- Sauerkraut

- Yogurt (with probiotics such as Lactobacillus or Acidophilus)

Travel and X-Rays

While traveling during pregnancy is relatively safe, there are potential risks. The official medical statement from the American Congress of Obstetricians and Gynecologists is that in the absence of obstetric or medical complications, pregnant women can observe the same precautions for air travel as the general population and can fly safely. But the fine print notes that in frequent flyers, the risks to the fetus from exposure to radiation may be higher. Since medical science does not have all the answers, especially as far as risks to the fetus are concerned, it's advisable to be informed about the possibilities in order to make the best decision for you and your growing family.

The obscure but notable risks of traveling while pregnant may include preterm birth or unforeseen emergencies such as bleeding complications. And of course, if you have specific medical conditions such as respiratory or cardiac diseases that might be exacerbated by the oxygen changes on a plane, or if you have a known risk for preterm labor, air travel should unequivocally be avoided. And if you're traveling to an area that requires specific vaccinations or medications, risks and benefits should be carefully weighed.

During pregnancy you also have an increased tendency toward blood clotting, and if you're continuing on any hormone therapy from assisted reproductive interventions, you may be at higher risk as well—beyond the already tenfold increase in the risk of *venous thromboembolism* (also called *deep venous thrombosis*)—when a blood clot breaks loose and travels through the blood. Cabin pressure and immobility while flying can be major contributors to this possibility. So, ladies, if you must fly, wear your support hose and walk around as much as possible.

If you have a choice in the matter, it's best to plan any necessary air travel for your second trimester. Risks of preterm birth are potentially minimized after twenty weeks, and after thirty-six weeks most airlines won't let you on a plane anyway, nor is it medically advisable to fly.

The real, research-based lowdown is that potential background radiation from cosmic rays—which, in truth, pass through you all the time, but are a little more intensive while flying—doesn't outweigh the normal statistics for things that would happen anyway. The main, grounded research is that you just shouldn't travel for a cumulative total of more than 150 hours while pregnant, as this would exceed the recommendation for fetal exposure to radiation. Airlines, for instance, monitor their employees as if they work at a nuclear facility.

The way I figure it, knowing that there is exposure at all, and knowing how these type of guidelines often change over time as more information and understanding emerges, I think it warrants serious evaluation as to whether to fly at all during this important time (most importantly during the first trimester). Perhaps planning a babymoon via road trip will suit you fine.

If you are going to fly, consider these pregnancy-safe foods and supplements to counteract in-flight radiation exposure:

Foods

- Olive Oil: Cold-pressed olive oil (extra virgin olive oil is better for you) helps protect the cell membranes from radiation.

- Chlorophyll-rich foods: This substance is found in alfalfa sprouts, celery, leafy greens, parsley, spirulina and chlorella (two micro-algae products), and wheatgrass. It helps the liver detoxify.

- Seaweeds: There are thousands of different types of seaweeds, but some of the most popular edible variations are dulse, kombu, nori, and wakame. They are easy to find at natural food stores, and can be mixed into soups and salads, or eaten by themselves. If you can't stomach eating seaweed, you can also find it powdered in capsules as a supplement. Also, it's important to also make sure the seaweed is sourced from areas that aren't known contaminated ocean waters. These are a known food to offset radiation exposure.

- Miso: A traditional Japanese seasoning produced by fermenting rye, beans, rice, or barley with salt and the fungus *kojikin*, has also been shown to help combat radiation exposure.

Other foods that help the body decrease the effects of radiation: apples, beets, broccoli, Brussels sprouts, cabbage, garlic, guavas, kale, nutritional yeast, onions, oranges, pineapple, plums, quince, and watercress.

In short, my advice to you when traveling while pregnant:

- Sport the support hose.
- Have a shot of wheatgrass and liberally use cold-pressed olive oil.
- Take a bolstered vitamin regimen throughout your trip.
- Enjoy gallivanting without a stroller while you still can!

Supplements

In addition to your prenatal, which should already include a B complex, consider adding:

- Calcium 1,000 mg
- Magnesium 500 mg
- Vitamin C with bioflavanoids 2 to 5 grams
- Vitamin E d-alpha-tocopherol about 900 IU per day

Notable mention: Selenium protects DNA from radiation damage and helps prevent damage to the skin surface too. You can get selenium directly from food by eating a daily dose of two cups of nettle infusion, one-half ounce of kelp, two ounces of cooked burdock root, or one cup of probiotic-rich yogurt. Many types of mushrooms also contain significant amounts of selenium.

Environmental Concerns

When it comes to exposure to environmental toxins and other concerns, I feel the same about pregnancy as I do about life in general. For better or worse, we don't live in—nor are we bringing a baby into—a bubble. We live in a modern world with modern concerns, and I suppose we can only hope and rely on our genetics and immune systems continuing to modify themselves enough to adapt and buffer the inevitable allergens and toxins that we're bound to encounter. So, it is unrealistic (and will probably drive you nuts) trying to avoid everything that has potential detriment to pregnancy. I'll present what the current literature says about some of the common things to avoid, and figuring that most of these are unavoidable for you, and I'll provide some ways to offset their potential infringement.

Cell Phones

It's true. Cell phones do emit electromagnetic radiation (EMR) and can affect you by increasing free radicals, which can lead to oxidative stress, which is basically an imbalance in your body's ability to detoxify or repair tissue damage.

Thankfully, as usual, nature has an answer. The bees heard the buzz, and one of the components of the honeybee hive, propolis, has been shown to be a potent free-radical scavenger and antioxidant. Other antioxidants that you may want to boost up on include Vitamin C (food sources include berries; broccoli; Brussels sprouts; cantaloupe; cauliflower; grapefruit; honeydew; kale; kiwi; mangoes; nectarines; orange; papaya; red, green, or yellow peppers; snow peas; sweet potato; strawberries; and tomatoes) and vitamin E (food sources include broccoli, carrots, chard, mustard and turnip greens, mangoes, nuts, papaya, pumpkin, red peppers, spinach, and sunflower seeds).

Ginkgo biloba has also been shown to prevent mobile phone-induced oxidative stress by preserving antioxidant enzyme activity in the brain. And don't store your phone in your bra or near your uterus!

Microwaves

It would seem that exposure to microwave radiation like fetal ultrasounds would be pretty innocuous. The risk that is attributed to normal exposure from these types of radiation is approximately 0.003 percent (thousands of times smaller than congenital risks independent of this exposure). Having said that, I always feel weird when I stand in front of a microwave, and as science is always evolving and uncovering potential risks. I still vote for minimizing your exposure. Stovetop popcorn is better anyway.

X-rays

X-rays are their own animal. Although it is preferable not to get an x-ray while pregnant, if a medical condition warrants it, your radiologist and physician will work to minimize the amount of radiation exposure you have.

Listeriosis

Listeria monocytogenes, the bacteria responsible for causing the infection known as listeriosis, has a rich history in obstetrics. Its namesake is Joseph Lister, the surgeon who realized that washing his hands between assisting deliveries minimized the mortality rates of women and their babies.

Now that we're clear on hand washing as a routine method of sanitation, we just have to watch out for processed and prepared foods infected with this bacterium. That's why hot dogs, deli meat, soft and unpasteurized cheeses, and smoked fish are always on the list of pregnancy no-nos.

The symptoms of listeriosis during pregnancy are difficult to distinguish from regular old pregnancy symptoms—fatigue and aches. So diagnosis and treatment (especially since Listeria's whole job is to protect itself from its host's immune response) can be difficult. Considering this, it's best to outright avoid known potential causes. If you do contract listeriosis, the usual course will be high-dose antibiotics and ultrasound monitoring of the baby.

Toxoplasmosis

Toxoplasmosis (from a parasite called Toxoplasma gondii) usually doesn't have any symptoms, but can occasionally present with flu-like symptoms such as swollen lymph nodes in your throat or armpits, body aches, and a temperature. If you are symptomatic, or if you think you may have been exposed to toxoplasmosis, you can get a blood test done to rule it out. The blood test can also check which type of antibody (if any) that you have: IgG antibodies means you've contracted this infection in the past and usually won't be infected again, whereas IgM antibodies indicate that it's a more recent infection (in the last eight weeks) and that your baby is at a slight, but potential, risk.

You can test the amniotic fluid, and the baby's blood can be drawn after birth as well. More than half of the babies who have been exposed to toxoplasmosis never have symptoms. However, sometimes symptoms can show up months or years later and affect their vision or hearing. Like most things in pregnancy, your baby is more susceptible to infection earlier on in your pregnancy.

If there is confirmed toxoplasmosis, some people turn to antibiotics to combat it.

The most common to least common sources for contracting toxoplasmosis are:

- Undercooked or raw meat
- Raw cured meat, such as salami or Parma ham
- Unpasteurized goats' milk
- Cat litter
- Soil

Avoid the activities and substances above, or at least wear gloves for changing litter and gardening.

Mold

Damp or water-damaged environments can result in a host of microbial growths of mold and bacteria and their by-products. This kind of exposure has been associated with a variety of respiratory and other health issues in moms and babies. If this is a problem in your home, it's pretty difficult to successfully eradicate. So, nesting during pregnancy may take on a new meaning—as you might want to look for a completely new place to live.

When to Announce Your Pregnancy

Your pregnancy announcement is a very personal decision. There is no right or wrong time. It's true that as your pregnancy goes along, there's less chance of miscarriage and more security in telling people. On the other hand, there can be something triumphant and liberating about making an announcement earlier on. Even though this may feel like a risk, indulging in your news and sharing with those who feel right to share with might feel incredibly supportive and give you more of the resources you need and deserve during the formative weeks.

There are many ways and times to let people know about your very personal development. You might prefer one-on-one discussions with those close to you, or you might fancy making a group announcement via social media, email, or another format. Regardless of how or who you tell, just think of each new person who knows as someone else you can potentially rant to about your pregnancy stuff.

When to announce at work can be a slightly more strategic matter. If you feel intimidated about the security of your position once you're pregnant, consult resources such as the Family and Medical Leave Act to know exactly what your rights are. I recommend approaching your boss or human resources department with a plan around your absence and reintegration. You may have come a long way to position yourself where you are in your company, and you might be perfectly capable of maintaining a work-life balance after your baby is born. Or, this might be a wonderful time to reevaluate what you'd like to do regarding your job. Babies have a funny way of helping you reprioritize.

Preparing Birth Announcements

If you're planning to send birth announcements to your friends and family, prepping them in advance and inserting pictures after baby is born can be a stress-relieving strategy later on. I've seen birth announcements from a simple email with the pertinent info (name, date of birth, birth weight, length) to glossy catalogs of the baby's first months and announcements on paper seeded with wildflowers that the recipient can then plant as an ongoing symbol of your little one's new growth. (You can check the resources section under baby announcements for leads on that last one.)

Checklist for Month Two

- If you haven't already had your first check-up, it's time (including the nuchal translucency test if that's part of your plan).
- Evaluate your decisions around genetic testing and schedule an amniocentesis or CVS, and nuchal translucency test if you're opting for any of these procedures.
- You may want to find some looser-fitting clothes at this stage to support your comfort, including a bra without underwire.

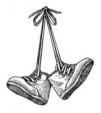

Month Three
Emerging

WEEK THIRTEEN

- Baby is 2.9 inches and .81 ounces.
- Head is now a third of the size of the body.
- Teeth are forming.
- The baby now has unique fingerprints.

WEEK FOURTEEN

- This is the start of your second trimester
- Baby is 3.4 inches and 1.5 ounces.
- Baby can suck his or her thumb.
- The lanugo, a thin layer of hair over the body, is keeping baby insulated.
- The baby's sex can be identified.
- Baby can hear the environment in your belly now too.

WEEK FIFTEEN

- Baby is 4 inches and 2.5 ounces.
- Baby can hiccup.
- All the joints and limbs are fully mobile.

....

WEEK SIXTEEN

- Baby is 4.6 inches and 3.5 ounces.
- You can probably feel baby moving now (but don't worry. It's also totally normal if you can't feel them yet).
- Your baby can grasp with fingers now.
- The body is filling out with more fat being deposited under the skin.
- Hair is appearing on the head along with eyebrows and eyelashes.

....

East-West Fetal Development

This month is represented by the Chinese Pericardium system. Your actual pericardium is the protective membrane around the heart, and as you build on the information you've gathered about your pregnancy, including test results and your personal experience of being pregnant, you may subsequently be even more trusting and confident in your pregnancy. Your heart may feel bolstered and open to newfound connection and joy—especially as some of the initial symptoms of the first trimester begin to recede.

In Chinese medicine, the Pericardium is the companion to the Heart; both systems are associated with the element of fire. During this phase, in response to your growing baby and increasing circulatory demands, your blood volume is increasing and may bring another round of heated symptoms such as heartburn. As with all of the phases of pregnancy, temper the ups and downs and trust that if the process itself is not fully enjoyable, the final result—your baby—will be. I feel confident that he or she will bring you a joy like none you've experienced.

Constipation and Heartburn

Constipation, heartburn, and hemorrhoids seem to be the triad of pregnancy, and this is the month when hints of any or all of these may creep in. (More on hemorrhoids in month five.) From a Chinese medicine perspective, these are all symptoms of stagnancy, which is not surprising if you think about growing a baby as "accumulating a baby." While your body is working hard to retain the baby, it's also retaining everything else. After all, accumulation is the opposite of elimination, and these other accumulations, namely constipation, often drive the heartburn and hemorrhoids. Focusing on the constipation can be a good start for managing or resolving the rest.

....

STOMACH-SOOTHING SLIPPERY ELM LOZENGES

Slippery elm contains *mucilage*, which means it turns into a gel when mixed with water. It also has potent antioxidants that relieve inflammation and stimulate increased mucus secretion in the stomach, which can coat or protect your stomach from acidity—hence helping heartburn.

Ingredients

> ¼ cup marshmallow root
>
> 1 tablespoon dried elderberries
>
> 1 cup water
>
> 2 tablespoons honey, divided equally
>
> ½ tablespoon slippery elm powder (plus some extra in a bowl for coating finished lozenges)

Directions

Add marshmallow root and elderberries to water, bring to a boil, and simmer with lid on for ten minutes. Pour 1 tablespoon honey and strained marshmallow root "tea" into a bowl.

In a separate bowl, slowly add remainder of honey to the slippery elm powder while stirring constantly with a wooden spoon. As you make this "dough," adjust the consistency by adding more slippery elm powder to firm it up, and begin to add the "tea" to moisten it, aiming for a smooth, not-too-sticky dough. Roll dough out to ¼-inch thickness and slice into discs about size of lozenges. I like to roll each lozenge in some extra slippery elm powder as well to keep them from sticking together. Dry lozenges on a plate for two days or bake at 250 degrees Fahrenheit for one hour.

....

Constipation

Whether you're backed up for days or hours, or just having difficulty moving your bowels, it's such an uncomfortable symptom to add to an already congested and bloated system. Constipation happens in about a third of pregnant women and, from a Western medicine point of view, is usually caused by rising progesterone levels, which affect intestinal motility.

Another culprit is iron supplementation. Even though iron is great to support your pregnancy, it can cause constipation. (See the anemia section for more details and tips on easily digestible sources of iron that can potentially help you avoid the supplement route.)

Hypothyroidism may also be an occasional cause of constipation during pregnancy. Make sure your thyroid has been evaluated, since the thyroid is the engine of the endocrine system and can experience changes during pregnancy.

Luckily, you may have some recourse from constipation. Most of the time, fluids, food, and exercise can restore normal bowel function. When you're constipated, your system isn't doing a great job of assimilating the nutrition you are taking in or distributing the nutrients, so it really helps to replenish your nutrients with fluids that contain electrolytes and easy-to-digest foods such as broths and porridges. (Refer to the Vitamin C-Rich Electrolyte Refresher and Boosted-Up Chicken stock recipes in month one, and the Ancient Grains Porridge recipe in month one.)

Heartburn

As the baby grows, the heart grows fonder, but heartburn also grows. Interestingly, baby's hair may be growing too! The same pregnancy hormones that contribute to heartburn by way of relaxing the esophageal sphincter (the muscles that keep food from going up the tube that connects the throat with the stomach) also promote fetal hair growth.

The occurrence of heartburn in pregnant women increases from 22 percent in the first trimester to 39 percent in the second trimester and then up to 72 percent in the third trimester. Basically, for most women, everything just gets exponentially more uncomfortable.

There are ways to deal with heartburn, and, like everything in pregnancy, we always try the lowest-impact intervention first. Start with diet changes (see the sidebar for some foods to add and others to avoid), and chew slowly

Morning Mini-Cleanse and Other Constipation Strategies

A great strategy to start with: every morning, drink a glass of warm water with the juice of half of a fresh-squeezed lemon. This is a validated folk remedy to promote the production of bile and help get the digestive system moving.

Next, take a look at your fiber intake. Plant fiber is technically not digestible, and it may seem weird to eat something inedible in order to help your digestion, but that's exactly the idea here. Plant fiber acts as a natural "scrub brush" for your intestines as it moves through your colon undigested. There are a lot of fiber-rich foods you can add to your diet, such as fruits, vegetables, nuts and seeds, legumes, and whole grains.

You can also consider bumping up your efforts with a psyllium husk supplement or a natural, pregnancy-safe laxative. However, be careful with laxatives. They also stimulate prostaglandins—fatty acids that enhance intestinal motility but also potentially soften your cervix and stimulate uterine contractions. Although you're possibly very uncomfortable with the constipation, it's best to ease into things and not shock your system. Regarding over-the-counter fiber products, obstetricians and gastroenterologists seem to favor the use of Citrucel, Colace, and Metamucil. Refraining from using castor oil. Check with your practitioner to make sure he or she agrees with this summary. Under no circumstances should you ever take laxative pills or mineral oils or receive colonic irrigation treatment during pregnancy. This can bring on early labor.

Exercise can be just as important as what you eat in getting your whole system "moving" again. Exercise tones your muscles and your cardiac system, and in the same way, it also helps stimulate the organs—especially the digestive organs. And, although you might not have a lot of energy right now, the good news is that it just takes a little movement to shift stagnancy in the body. Walking is a great place to start. A gentle yoga class is another fantastic recourse. Depending upon your normal pre-pregnancy exercise routine (and the input of your practitioner, of course), you might also consider a more rigorous yoga class, hiking, dancing, simple stretching exercises, or swimming. The Internet is rife with pregnancy exercise video options.

Of course, you always want to listen to your body and never push yourself past the point of comfort or safety—while pregnant or not.

and thoroughly (this stimulates digestive secretions to help your stomach more optimally process food and minimize the secretion of unnecessary acid).

If changing your eating habits doesn't do the trick, the next line of defense can be Western interventions including Milk of Magnesia, calcium carbonate-based antacids (these rarely have adverse effects; plus they've been shown to be beneficial for the prevention of high blood pressure and pre-eclampsia). If you've been diligent with diet and lifestyle changes, heartburn symptoms are unrelenting and you're still seeking temporary relief, histamine H2-receptor antagonists (also known as H2 blockers or acid reducers) are sometimes used, and if it's really, really bad, in severe instances, proton pump inhibitors can be prescribed, but as ever, it's advisable to avoid drugs during pregnancy if possible. Be sure to check in with your physician about appropriate options. Although you might not be able to completely get rid of heartburn, it may be possible to at least minimize the discomfort.

NOTE: If you are one of the few who has been prescribed medications to control nausea and vomiting, these can cause heartburn.

Things to Avoid to Minimize Heartburn

- anti-inflammatory drugs
- caffeine
- carbonated drinks
- chocolate
- citrus
- dairy (except for probiotic-rich yogurt)
- greasy and spicy foods
- garlic
- mint
- mustard
- onions
- refined flour
- tomatoes
- vinegar
- lying down within three hours after eating

....

MY HEART BURNS FOR YOU

It can be challenging to feel like you're supporting your nutrition during a time when you might not feel like eating, or wondering what you *can* eat without too many repercussions. Since it's advisable to eat small meals and snacks throughout the day to minimize the burden on your stomach, here's a recipe that fits the bill in size and contains nutrient and protein-rich ingredients that are also soothing for digestion.

By the way, the term "carat" evolved from the use of carob seeds as weight units for measuring gold, and carob is worth its weight in gold if it helps you feel better at this stage of your pregnancy.

Ingredients

¼ cup carob powder

1 teaspoon slippery elm powder

2 tablespoons sesame seed butter (tahini)

1 teaspoon green powder (such as spirulina or chlorella)

1 tablespoon honey

1 teaspoon chia seeds

Directions

Combine everything in a bowl and mix. Roll into small balls (about a tablespoon worth). Eat one or two a day. You can keep the rest in the fridge.

....

Things to Add to Minimize Heartburn

- Carob powder (see My Heart Burns for You recipe in this chapter)
- Magnesium-rich foods such as avocado, dry-roasted almonds, halibut, kelp, kidney beans, lentils, spinach, wheat bran, wheat germ, and yogurt with live cultures.
- Probiotics
- Zinc

Any of the previous concoctions for constipation may also help with heartburn.

Thyroid

The thyroid is the engine of the body, the crux of hormone regulation, and the gland at the core of metabolism. Pregnancy makes a lot of increased demands on your body, and it's no exception that the thyroid is working overtime—especially in regard to stimulating enzymes that help metabolize nutrients and oxidation of glucose. (Even though sugar often gets a bad rap, this form of sugar is one of the building blocks for your baby.)

To process all of this glucose, you end up increasing your oxygen uptake and basal metabolic rate (BMR). During pregnancy, there is a 20 to 30 percent increase BMR, and with this increase, symptoms that mimic hyperthyroidism can arise such as fatigue, a feeling of anxiety, sweating, heat sensitivity, warm skin, shortness of breath, edema and higher pulse rate. It's often difficult to differentiate between symptoms of normal pregnancy and a state of hyperthyroidism. True hyperthyroidism only occurs in .08 percent of pregnancies, though.

Your continued quick lesson in endocrinology is that there are two thyroid hormones: thyroxine (T4) and triiodothyronine (T3). One reason these hormones get stimulated during pregnancy is because the increased

....

SOOTHING THYME AND HONEY DIGESTIF

Thyme has a therapeutic effect on inflammatory conditions, especially in the digestive tract, including heartburn. This is a delicious, refreshing cold-brewed tea that you can make in big batches to always have on hand.

Directions
Pour 4 cups of warm (but not boiling—you don't want to destroy the important volatile plant oils) water over ½ cup of fresh thyme and ½ cup of honey. Stir and let cool. Add 2 cups of fresh-squeezed lemon juice to the thyme water. Mix. Pour over ice and enjoy.

....

estrogen of pregnancy stimulates the liver to double up the amount of thyroid hormone-binding proteins (TBG) it produces. As you can imagine from the word "binding," the hormones are occupied and not available, or "free." So, the body pumps out more of the aptly named "thyroid stimulating hormone" (TSH) to compensate. Your baby also secretes thyroid hormones around twelve weeks. That's why it's really important to assess a baseline and late pregnancy thyroid test and look at the "free" or circulating amounts of thyroid hormones. Note that lab ranges already take into account that thyroid levels are bound (pun intended) to be a little higher during pregnancy.

Additionally, calcitonin, which manages the calcium level in your blood, is also produced by the thyroid cells. When it's elevated it removes calcium from the blood and stores it in your bones and kidney cells. Estrogen (which naturally increases during pregnancy) can influence this process, which in turn inhibits calcium from being released and helps conserve your bone density.

For the most part, the body adjusts to all of these changes and acquires a new equilibrium, but these metabolic adjustments pose a problem when there is an existing autoimmune thyroid disease, hypothyroidism, or inadequate iodine in one's diet, and since the thyroid hormones are so prevalent in the body, they can have a swathe of adverse effects on a developing baby. It is important to concertedly manage thyroid issues during pregnancy.

Please note that iodine should not be thrown at any thyroid issue. It can actually throw off the thyroid even more and contribute to an increase in autoimmune thyroid issues. It reduces an enzyme called *thyroid peroxidase* (TPO), which is essential for normal thyroid hormone production. So, if you have the "right" kind of iodine-deficient hypothyroid condition and you're supplementing with iodine (or dosing up on seaweed), just be sure to recheck your thyroid labs every four to six weeks.

Nasal Congestion, Snoring, and Nosebleeds

Barring a cold, nasal congestion is just a phlegmy aspect of pregnancy that comes with growing a huge mass of human. It's called *pregnancy rhinitis*, which simply translates to "pregnancy-induced runny nose." If this inflammatory condition persists, the delicate membranes of your nose can be more susceptible to actual infection. The congestion can also, of course, impair your breathing, and in addition to being a nuisance, fluids accumulate in your upper respiratory tract particularly when you're lying down. So snoring becomes an issue too.

On the other spectrum, throughout pregnancy, your blood volume and estrogen increase, which both can lead to increased blood flow in the membranes of your nose, leading to a susceptibility toward nosebleeds even from minor irritations. If you already tend toward nasal irritations or infections, they may worsen during pregnancy. If this is not a general concern for you, a runny or even bloody nose may still be part of your pregnancy repertoire. Perhaps an opportunity to carry around stylish handkerchiefs?

The Reality behind Feeling Fat

It tends to be confusing for women that, within the first few weeks of finding out they're pregnant, they seem to already need maternity clothes. Not to fret! This is mostly due to a normal initial accumulation of fluids due to rapid hormone changes and the immediate needs of the newly growing baby. In the second trimester, fluid retention will typically subside and be replaced by tauter, more proportional, baby-related growth.

In general you can expect to gain the most weight in your stomach (obviously), hips, back, and upper thighs during pregnancy, since these areas are where estrogen (which is produced in high quantities during pregnancy to help protect and secure your pregnancy) is distributed and stored in fat tissue. Set your expectations now about your changing body.

It's true that throughout your pregnancy you will gain weight, and for a very good reason. There are a lot of factors at work. The placenta can alter your blood sugar and stimulate weight gain. Other components of weight gain include protein, fat, water, and minerals that are deposited in the fetus, placenta, amniotic fluid, uterus, mammary glands, blood, and adipose tissue. (The adipose tissue is what we commonly call "fat," and that's where a lot of this important stuff is stored.) Most of this weight gain can be lost when you and your baby don't need the intense nutrients anymore. Think of pregnancy as your body's way of storing up for a long winter. Basically, your body is conserving what you need for pregnancy, birth, and breastfeeding.

Just make sure you're experiencing the type of weight gain that is ultimately supportive for you and your baby, because it is also true that obesity is an increasing problem—especially in the United States—and can contribute to risk factors for pregnancy, birth, and the baby, such as preeclampsia, hypertension, gestational diabetes, the need for labor induction, or a baby that's large for her gestational age, which increases the likelihood of having a caesarean section. If weight was a pre-existing issue for you, and your pregnancy weight gain is already way outside the boundaries of average, now would be a great time to get going on a more supportive eating and exercise routine for you and your baby. Your habits will most likely become your children's habits too.

Having said that, weight gain in pregnancy is like growth in children: there's a wide range of normal. Humans are actually the most diverse species on the planet—from Pygmies to Samoans. Regardless, it's never comfortable to feel like you're outside the "norm" in your pregnancy. The normal rule of thumb is about two to four pounds of weight gain in the first trimester and just about a pound per week in the second and third trimesters, with slight adjustments to these numbers if you were either underweight or overweight when you conceived. For twins, the general guideline is a total gain of about thirty-seven to fifty-five pounds.

Every pregnant woman I've ever met has one thing in common: she hates when people guess (wrong) how far along she is in her pregnancy—particularly when she has some months to go and is told that she looks like she's "ready to pop." During the last months of pregnancy, the impacts of weight gain and stamina can be challenging.

Some people believe that women should not be weighed at all during pregnancy, since the "number" can produce unnecessary anxiety without any real added benefit. If you're eating well, have a healthy exercise regimen, and baby is meeting regular growth expectations via measurements and ultrasounds, you can probably safely assume that you are gaining the right amount of weight for you and your baby. But if your underlying blood sugar isn't stable, you can be doing all the right things without getting the right results. Manage your blood-sugar stability by eating small, protein-based meals throughout the day—balanced with whole grains, vegetables, and moderate amounts of fruit—along with managing any clinical aspects of blood sugar changes. Check out the section on gestational diabetes for more in-depth information on this topic.

Eating and weight are usually sensitive issues for women, with many emotional layers and habits to contend with. Don't feel bad if you have the best intentions but are having difficulty articulating them. If you're feeling very stressed about weight gain, consider seeking help from a nutritionist or a psychologist who (especially together) can help you set reasonable and healthy goals. You know the saying "It takes a village to raise a child"? Well, it can also take one to get through a pregnancy.

And one more thing: if you're worried about the idea of birthing a really big baby as a result of excessive weight gain, I've rarely seen a woman whose birth canal could not accommodate her baby. The exception to this is excessive growth caused by out-of-the-norm blood sugar or more serious genetic complications. Contrary to popular belief, "birthing hips" are not visible to the casual observer. Even if you are petite, what is of relevance in birth is the internal pelvic outlet. This loosens and opens to accommodate your baby, and frankly, in the throes of birth, you're really not able to differentiate between six pounds and eight pounds. It's a lot of baby, either way, but you get through it.

Remember, your body is doing what it needs to do to support a healthy pregnancy and grow a baby that it is designed to accommodate.

The Ins and Outs of Intercourse

Just like in your normal love life, sexual desire can go every which way during pregnancy. There are more hormones flying around and increased blood perfusion into reproductive tissue, which could account for many women's increased sex drive at certain stages in their pregnancy. This is a time of not only heightened physical sensitivity, but emotional sensitivity as well. Listening to your body and doing what feels right for you can become its own source of pleasure. Whatever the origin of your desires, if you're in the mood, it can be confusing, disappointing, and painful if you or your partner feels nervous about acting on your impulses. Just like you, your partner may be having a new process around his or her sexuality. Often, partners feel that they will be injuring the baby, hurting you, or doing something morally inappropriate if you have intercourse.

This is an important juncture to communicate together about any deep concerns, thoughts, or judgments, and it's also an opportunity to navigate the many disparities that arise in relationships and in parenting. It is a place that can be a catalyst for reconciling your view of yourself as both a mother and an intimate partner. It may help to know that, barring any conditions that may warrant abstaining from sex at certain stages, sex is a safe and healthy way to continue to bond throughout a pregnancy. Conditions that you would want to look out for would include existing risk of miscarriage or preterm labor threat, placenta previa, unexplained vaginal bleeding, or if your practitioner has recommended abstaining for another reason.

Other Facts to Help Quell Your Concerns about Sex during Pregnancy

First, let's talk about the actual anatomy going on here. Know that your baby is completely contained within the amniotic sac and will not be exposed to any of the sexual fluids. There is also a thick mucus plug that seals the cervix during pregnancy to guard against infection or anything else entering the uterus. Neither the penis nor the semen comes into contact with the baby during sex.

I would surmise that if the baby is privy to anything, it's probably the unconscious feeling of their parents loving and caring for each other. As a matter of fact, oxytocin is released during a woman's orgasm, which is the same "bonding hormone" that helps facilitate not only bonding between partners, but also bonding with the baby after birth. It's notable that oxytocin is also released during warm touch and prolonged gazing into each other's eyes. So cuddling might satiate you if sex doesn't appeal right now.

Rest assured that unless there is already a threat, sex does not cause miscarriages. Miscarriages are typically due to chromosomal abnormalities or unknown causes unrelated to sex. Oral sex is also safe during pregnancy, but your partner should refrain from blowing any air into your vagina. Although it's very rare, this can cause an air embolism, which can be life threatening during pregnancy.

The primary concern about anal sex during pregnancy is the spread of infection to the vagina. So, be sure to be cognizant of hygiene if this is in your repertoire.

If you need extra inspiration, think about this: by virtue of the new mechanics of sex during pregnancy, you might even find yourself making up new positions with each other. This can be an exciting time to expand your sensuality in whatever way feels right for you.

Cold and Flu Facts and Prevention

Pregnant women have about the same amount of colds and flus as nonpregnant women, but because your body's resources are a bit preoccupied, you may be at risk for more complications from a "simple" cold or flu than you normally would. Specifically, your T-helper cells (which mediate part of your immunity) are slightly suppressed during pregnancy, your heart is working harder, and your oxygen uptake is a little lower. This means you may be more likely to get pneumonia or, in extreme circumstances, experience premature delivery. However, Chinese medicine also recognizes that during pregnancy you are storing up energy in your Kidney system, and the Kidneys are the root of immunity. So many women's overall health actually greatly improves during pregnancy.

A general Western medical recommendation is to receive the flu shot during pregnancy. The flu shot is a guess, albeit an educated guess, on which strain of virus will be most prevalent during a particular season. Viruses tend to mutate differently in everyone's systems. So, the flu shot may or may not be an effective combatant for you.

Additionally, it's a bit of a misnomer that the flu shot prevents the flu. Actually, it is designed to shorten the duration of your flu symptoms by only a few days and perhaps lessen the severity of the impact. Having said this, if you are severely immune compromised (as Western medicine conjectures you are during pregnancy), it's worth doing what you can to minimize your risks of infection. If this doesn't seem like it applies to you, or doesn't appeal to you, it may be worth considering allowing your own immune system to respond to the assault of the season to set the precedent of a protective mechanism for this and subsequent strains. As ever, check with your health-care provider about your specifics.

I tend to be of the school of thought that in order to best treat yourself without risking harm, you should always try to treat yourself first with food or plant-based medicines. But healthy doesn't just mean medication free; it means making the most well rounded and healthiest decision for you and your baby. So trust yourself and those on your healthcare team.

....

IMMUNE CIDER

Many of the ingredients in this recipe are natural immune tonics with antibacterial and anti-inflammatory properties.

Ingredients

3 tablespoons grated horseradish root

3 tablespoons grated ginger root

3 tablespoons chopped fresh parsley

One medium onion, peeled and finely chopped

One whole head of garlic, peeled and finely chopped

1 cayenne, habanero, or Serrano pepper, finely chopped (optional)

Raw, organic, unfiltered apple cider vinegar, to fill jar

You will also need two large glass jars with tight-fitting lids.

Directions

Place all chopped ingredients into a glass jar. Pour apple cider vinegar over the mixture all the way to the top of the jar. Make sure all ingredients are covered and no air is trapped, and secure the lid tightly. Allow to soak for two weeks (or longer) in the fridge. Drain the liquid into a fresh clean jar. Discard the solids. Keep tonic refrigerated. It will last this way for a few months.

Ways to use your concoction:

1. Take 1 to 2 tablespoons as needed to stave off a cold or flu.

2. Make a "hot toddy" with your immune cider by adding a tablespoon or two to hot water with some honey and lemon juice, to taste.

3. Add it to salad dressings.

....

If you do get sick, just a quick note: as nasal decongestants *do not* have a lower risk to the fetus than oral medications, you may want to investigate some over-the-counter herbal remedies designed specifically for pregnancy, such as WishGarden's tincture line (see resource section). You can also try a simple face steam over a bowl of hot water, with a few drops of eucalyptus essential oil added to clear out the nose. I am partial to the Immune Cider recipe below, and the Stomach-Soothing Slippery Elm Lozenge recipe on page 89 also works as a pregnancy-safe, soothing remedy to alleviate inflammation and discomfort.

Strep Throat

Even though you may be healthy, immune-system changes during pregnancy can make you feel a bit like a petri dish. If your throat is scratchy or burning, and you're having difficulty swallowing (especially if accompanied by a fever), you'll want to do a strep test to confirm the culture before jumping to conclusions about your sore throat, but if you do have strep, the typical coarse is antibiotics. You can also introduce the remedies in the cold and flu section above to contribute to getting better.

By the way, this is completely unrelated to Group B streptococcus, which we'll talk about in month nine.

Fifth Disease

Fifth disease, named this, by the way, because it's fifth in a list of historical skin diseases. It looks like a red rash on your face, and is caused by parvovirus B19 and spread via respiratory secretions such as coughing and sneezing. Although it's very contagious (and sometimes the baby does catch it), it's usually not a problem for you or your baby, and since it's a virus, there's really nothing to do for it other than work on natural immune-building strategies and rest. It usually self-resolves within ten days.

How to Quit Smoking

You may or may not be surprised to hear that about 10 percent of women smoke during pregnancy. The primary risks with this are delivering prematurely and low birth-weight babies, which can impair baby's own immunity and resources for beginning the life ahead of him. If you've tried to quit in the past and feel discouraged, the good news is that, statistically, the more times you've tried to quit, the more successful you're likely to be now. I like to think of smoking less as an addiction and more as one of many various habits that we develop in our life. It is less about withdrawing—since once you stop smoking, the nicotine in your blood immediately begins to decrease and recedes completely in about a week—and more about repatterning. This can be a great opportunity not only to get healthier, but also to possibly explore and develop some new hobbies or habits.

In Chinese medicine, we adhere to the idea of stimulating your inherent ability to take care of yourself. So most of the tools I recommend are based on implementing diet and lifestyle support that you can do at home to help you in your process and long-term health. As an addition to this, I do highly recommend acupuncture, which has lots of research behind its role in effectively helping manage and curb addictions (and is safe during pregnancy). One of acupuncture's mechanisms of action is that it produces endorphins, which can be good assistance during the initial period of cravings.

Here's an outline of what I give women at my clinic to get them started.

Preparing

On the day that you're ready to quit (hopefully this corresponds with having an acupuncture visit scheduled), clean out all of your ashtrays and throw away all cigarettes. You're about to get busy.

I suggest that you identify a buddy for support outside of the times that you will be seen by your acupuncturist—someone to communicate with you during any rough patches.

Grocery Shopping and Cooking Tips

Miso soup can help neutralize and clear the blood of nicotinic acid and fortify the blood sugar.

Add magnesium-rich foods like carrots, citrus fruits, dark leafy greens, legumes, pregnancy-preferred seafood, and whole grains to help alkalize the body and neutralize the acidity that smoking causes. People with a body pH of 7 and above show a decreased desire for tobacco.

Cook with turmeric to help neutralize cancer-causing agents. NOTE: turmeric is best utilized in the body when cooked for long periods of time such as in a slow-simmered soup or stew.

Eat baked Asian pears to help moisten and soothe the lungs.

Foods to Avoid

Avoid oxalic-acid-forming foods like chocolate, cooked spinach, and ruta-baga that bind up magnesium in the body.

Avoid white sugar and white flour products such as breads, candy, cookies, pastries, and soda, as well as sugary juices, which deplete nutrients and create an acidic condition in the body—which can aggravate your cravings. A caveat that I like to add to this is that if short-term sugar intake soothes your nerves as you're denying yourself those initial smokes, go ahead and indulge for a week or two, and then you can worry about reducing your sugar.

Avoid deep-fried foods and margarines, as they generate inflammatory and oxidative reactions in the body.

Cleanse and Supplements

Pregnancy is not a good time to do cleanses. Just focus on eating as cleanly as you can (fresh vegetable juices, lots of leafy greens, broths, soups and stews, and whole foods versus refined foods), and you can also supplement with:

Vitamin C: 1,000 mg, four times a day. Your body is severely depleted of vitamin C by smoking. As an antioxidant, vitamin C is instrumental in neutralizing the toxic by-products of smoking. See the section on vitamin C for more specifics on foods to boost up on and see the recipe for the Electrolyte Refresher in month one's recipes.

If you must, herbal cigarettes or nicotine gum or patches can help with the transition as well.

Exercise and Relaxation

Get physical: Physical activity can help distract you from your cravings and reduce their intensity. Try to walk for thirty minutes a day during the first few weeks of quitting. If you're unable to get out of the house or your office, try deep knee bends, push-ups, squats, or walking up and down a set of stairs a few times.

Get relaxed: Practice relaxation techniques. Coping with your cravings can be very stressful. In addition, smoking may have been the very way that you coped with stress and anxiety in the first place. Replace your stress-coping mechanism with a healthy alternative by practicing relaxation techniques. These include deep-breathing exercises, hypnosis, massage, visualization, and yoga. You can also download guided imagery exercises online. See the resource section for a reputable source for guided imagery.

Hydration

Drink at least ten to fifteen glasses of liquid a day, including water, soup, or broths. Hydration is essential for replenishing the lungs and counteracting the effects of the drying and acidifying effects of smoking.

Distraction

When cravings strike, distract yourself with healthy alternatives to smoking such as:

- Breathing deeply for a few minutes to increase oxygen in the body
- Going for a walk
- Munching on carrot and celery sticks (even better to munch on the ginger carrot pickles in month two's recipe section)
- Chewing sugar-free gum
- Sucking or chewing on cinnamon sticks, licorice sticks, mints, or toothpicks
- Crafting, drawing, knitting, or other busywork that occupies your hands
- Doing lunges, push-ups, or squats until the cravings pass
- Using ear seeds (which your acupuncturist can place for you) to help with withdrawal symptoms
- Going to the movies or other entertaining environments where smoking is prohibited

Emotional Support

Don't hesitate to call on your friends and family for support. Talk about your struggles. If you need deeper emotional support around your process, seek out a therapist to help you recognize and reorganize your patterns around smoking and assist you in creating new, more supportive habits.

....

BAKED ASIAN PEAR TO SOOTHE A SINGED THROAT

Core out an Asian pear, wrap in tinfoil, and bake at 450 degrees Fahrenheit for about forty-five minutes or until soft. Eat an Asian pear every night before bed to help rid your lungs of phlegm and soothe coughing.

....

Checklist for Month Three

Essential

- Schedule monthly prenatal visits.
- Decide when and how to announce your pregnancy.
- Begin planning maternity leave.

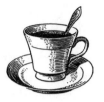

Month Four
Assimilating

WEEK SEVENTEEN

- Baby is 5.1 inches and 5.9 ounces.
- Cartilage is turning to bone.

WEEK EIGHTEEN:

- Baby is 5.6 inches and 6.7 ounces.
- There are noticeable movements now.

WEEK NINETEEN:

- Baby is 6 inches and 8.5 ounces.
- The five senses are starting to develop.
- The *vernix caseosa* (a waxy substance coating the skin) is formed.

WEEK TWENTY:

- Baby is 6.5 inches and 10.2 ounces.
- He or she is increasing the consumption of amniotic fluid.
- The placenta is fully formed.

East-West Fetal Development

This month is associated with the Chinese Triple Burner System. This is an abstract system in Chinese medicine, with the closest Western correlative being the circulation of fluids throughout the body and the idea of metabolism. This concept is very pertinent during this particular fetal development stage, as baby begins to swallow amniotic fluid, which now passes through her own digestive system and is processed into her working kidneys, then excreted back into the amniotic fluid as urine.

The amount of amniotic fluid can help indicate if the baby is potentially having any difficulty with the swallowing reflex before birth. By the time the baby is ready to be born, she'll be consuming about fifteen ounces of amniotic fluid each day. This, along with baby's working taste buds, means there's a lot for both of you to digest at this stage. There is even research suggesting that what you eat during pregnancy is passed into the amniotic fluid in the form of a flavor that may influence what your child finds palatable later on. So, like the increasing demands for your own output and baby's inner workings, the system that's most at work this month is all about taking in nutrients and churning them into energy.

Vaginal Fluids and Infections

Okay, we've all heard the simile that a woman's vagina is like a flower, but I don't think we like to think of it as a garden of flora and microbes! During pregnancy, estrogen is at an all-time high, and estrogen contributes to glycogen (a carbohydrate that breaks down to glucose, or sugar) being deposited in the epithelial cells that line the vaginal walls. Glycogen also gets metabolized into lactic acid, which is what acidifies the vagina. This is a long-winded way of saying there's normal discharge from pregnancy, and there's also a predisposition to a higher content of acid in your vagina, which can set you up for susceptibility to infection.

It's always a bit disconcerting to have anything going on out of the ordinary *down there*, and it's important to differentiate between normal changes versus something that might indicate an infection or any other complication. Below is an outline of the typical things to look out for during pregnancy and what they might mean. For anything out of the ordinary, you should definitely consult your care provider.

....

A SOOTHING VAGINAL SOAK AND SEAL

Saline Soak

Oddly, saline doesn't sting as much as regular water. Mix 1 teaspoon of salt with 4 cups of water, soak for ten minutes, and dry off well (but gently). Then use the topical powder below.

Clay and Goldenseal Dust

> 1 cup white clay (if you can't find white clay, regular cosmetic clay will do)
>
> ½ cup cornstarch
>
> 2 tablespoons myrrh powder*
>
> 1 tablespoon goldenseal powder*

*See resource section for a myrrh and goldenseal powder source.

Sift all ingredients together and dust on as needed.

Chinese medicine also has a wonderful topical remedy called *Yin Care Herbal Wash* (see resource section).

....

Leukorrhea

This is a viscous, white, odorless discharge without any other symptoms that, like the general vaginal discharge described above, comes from the increased estrogen being converted by Lactobacillus acidophilus (that's why acidophilus is a good suppository in the vagina for yeast infections) into glycogen. It's really normal to have this type of discharge during pregnancy, and your only real solution is panty liners. This secretion also perks up later in pregnancy to help flush the vagina and contribute to preventing infection as you get closer to birth.

Vulvar Pruritis

This is characterized by itching with pain, burning, and tenderness. It can be due to the pH changes in the vaginal environment or from vitamin A, B, or B12 deficiency. See the Anatomy of a Prenatal Vitamin section for foods that are chock-full of these nutrients, and then soak and seal with the wash and topical salve in the following recipe.

Easy Anti-Inflammatory Eating Plan for Candida

A wide range of issues have been linked to Candida, including depression, digestive irregularities, poor concentration, chronic fatigue, thyroid disorders, and even multiple sclerosis—and, of course, systemic inflammation. Sustained inflammation in the body can have serious and far-reaching consequences.

Vulvovaginal candidiasis usually presents as a thick, white, cottage cheese-like discharge without a significant odor. You may also have other skin irritations on your body or some noticeable digestive changes. However, these kinds of changes can be difficult to differentiate from the other effects of pregnancy. Dealing with *Candida albicans,* the primary infecting agent of Candida (more commonly known as a yeast infection), is usually based on a diet-driven strategy.

In Chinese medicine we look for the root cause of an issue. Where did this overgrowth come from? Certainly not just sugar, which is so often to blame for Candida. It is more probable that the origin is a digestive system that doesn't effectively break down, assimilate, and appropriately eliminate what it's taking in. A strong digestive system should be able to tolerate moderate amounts of sugar and other Candida "culprits" such as gluten, starchy vegetables, and dairy. So, I don't advocate a typical "eliminate sugar forever and everything else you normally eat" diet to control Candida. Instead, I'm going to outline a super simple strategy for you to repair, strengthen, and build your digestion for long-term normal eating that will help you rid Candida.

Once you've made a shift in your eating habits, you will be able to return to some of your favorite indulgences eventually—in moderation. On the backdrop of the new foundation you will create, they won't impact you as negatively as they once may have.

I'm an advocate of introducing foods rather than heavily eliminating them—especially during pregnancy, when the goal is often simply to eat whatever you can to make it through. When you present the right stuff to your system, the unhealthier cravings naturally become less severe. Initially we tend to crave foods that fuel our imbalances, but when your system is back in balance, it will do a good job of being attracted to things that are good for it—or at least that it can tolerate well.

A food plan should be individualized medicine based on your immune system, digestive system, etc. The following is a general outline of a typical anti-inflammatory eating strategy, which is the crux of optimizing your digestion. You can also ask your provider to order an IgG food allergy test from The Great Plains Laboratory, Inc. to identify your particular sensitivities to approximately ninety foods that are common triggers for hypersensitivity. It might help you hone in more specifically on which foods to eliminate to best support you.

The main thing to focus on is eating five small protein-based meals throughout the day. This keeps your blood sugar stable and helps to optimize metabolism. Remember that protein is not just meat. Think of other protein sources such as almonds, walnuts, hummus, or quinoa.

Next, focus on incorporating good-quality fats and oils—avocado, coconut oil, sesame oil, and olive oil—and cook with anti-inflammatory spices such as turmeric, rosemary, cumin, and cinnamon.

Slow-cooked foods are the easiest to digest, because some of the work of breaking down the food has already been done for you. Bonus: one-pot cooking makes elaborate meal planning a lot easier. It's also great preparation for cooking for baby down the road.

And yes, of course at first you'll want to minimize if not entirely eliminate sugar for a few weeks just to give yourself a jumpstart.

If I had to pick one supplement to add to the mix, I'd choose a probiotic. Please note that antibiotics and anti-inflammatory agents (ironically) can contribute to Candida.

Successful dietary changes usually require preparation so that you're ready and equipped to support your new change. So, draw on some of the principles and food above to create a personalized menu for yourself, map out your upcoming days, and figure out how you're going to incorporate your new eating habits into your schedule. And go stock up on groceries!

Eating away at inflammation is easy. You just have to be diligent. Give yourself about four to six weeks before assessing how you're feeling and whether or not the changes you've made are working for you.

Bacterial Vaginosis

Bacterial Vaginosis (BV) is a distinct discharge characterized by its thin grayish or white color and generally fishy odor, especially after intercourse. It's not typically accompanied by itching or burning. This infection is caused by a proliferation of organisms, including *Gardnerella vaginalis*.

The absence of Lactobacilli in the vagina is a specific feature of BV, so using probiotics can be an effective solution for protecting against the infection, as it can restore the normal vaginal flora. BV is associated with the risk of premature labor due to causing rupture of the membranes, and research on probiotics has shown that they can improve the chances of having a healthy full-term pregnancy by interfering with the inflammatory pathway that leads to premature rupture of the membranes and thereby premature labor. Probiotics have also been shown to promote healthy embryo development. Basically I'm pro probiotics for this situation.

Trichomoniasis

Trichomoniasis is a sexually transmitted disease involving the protozoan *Trichomonas vaginalis*. Trichomoniasis can be insidious in that it's often asymptomatic. Sometimes, it can be detected by itching, burning, redness, or soreness of your vaginal tissue, discomfort with urination, or a thin discharge with an unusual smell that can be clear, white, yellowish, or greenish. This type of infection can also be associated with premature rupture of membranes and preterm delivery. If you suspect that you have it, it's important to seek treatment guidance from your care provider right away.

Dysuria and Cystitis

Dysuria, or pain during urination, is usually felt externally when the urine touches the vulva. In contrast, internal dysuria, or pain inside the urethra, is usually a sign of cystitis.

Both of the above typically indicate a urinary tract infection, and any of these symptoms should trigger a visit to your care provider for further evaluation.

Overall Solutions

Besides getting appropriate consultation around any questionable symptoms, with any of the above symptoms you should wear loose-fitting clothing and cotton underwear, and keep yourself clean and dry.

Additionally, due to the acidic aspect of most vaginal infections, alkalizing your diet is usually a great approach to combating unwanted infections. (Following guidelines in the Easy Anti-Inflammatory Eating Plan for Candida sidebar section will take care of alkalizing you.)

Most inflammation of the vagina occurs because the vaginal flora has been altered by the introduction of pathogens or changes in the vaginal environment. Probiotics are a great solution for almost every woman with any of the above symptoms, or just as a pregnancy infection preventative.

Rearranging Your Sleeping Position

You may be sending S.O.S. signals for getting a good night's sleep and wondering what position you should be sleeping in or what might facilitate some rest. The truth is, although it's typically recommended to start sleeping on your side (and preferably the left side to promote maximum blood flow more easily through the heart—this has to do with the anatomy between the cardiac iliac artery and vein), as you progress in your pregnancy, your body will be your best guide as to when that's the best position.

Basically, you'll just know when you can't sleep on your back anymore. You'll know because you'll get dizzy or out of breath. It can be challenging to retrain sleeping positions away from what you're used to. Start out in the textbook position, and you'll just end up how you end up, and adjust as needed. You can also experiment with propping yourself up more, always bearing in mind that *sleeping is more valuable than not sleeping.* So get it in whatever position you can.

Childbirth Classes

Childbirth classes differ in their focus and philosophies, but they all have the same goal in mind: getting you through your birth with more choices and options for optimal positioning and preparation. I've attended a reasonable amount of births, and what strikes me most is that women have a natural instinct for what they want and need in the throes of labor. You can primarily rely on your intuition, but if you'd like to give your intuition more fodder to draw from and involve your partner as well, here's a basic review of some of the common types of childbirth classes out there:

What Is a Holistic Pediatrician?

If you're reading this book, you're probably at least curious if not already actively implementing some holistic aspects into the health of your pregnancy, and you may be interested in extending some of these values to your child's pediatric care too. Currently, over 6 percent of children are consuming medications primarily for behavioral disorders such as attention deficit hyperactivity disorder (ADHD). There is an increasing body of studies linking poor diet to the root cause of erratic changes in a child's blood sugar and brain chemistry and, subsequently, their behavioral and learning patterns.

It might seem easier and less daunting to experiment with your own health than to think about treating your child solely with herbal or nutrition-based medicine. I think the best of both worlds is a holistic pediatrician—someone who is grounded in sound Western medical advice and can collaborate with you on controversial issues such as vaccines and antibiotics. Additionally, you can talk with your pediatrician—holistic or otherwise—about simply using your visits for diagnostic information in order to help you come up with an appropriate integrative treatment strategy. If you are choosing to approach your child's health primarily with natural remedies, you can utilize a pediatrician for a sound diagnosis and to help monitor your child's progress and make sure you don't miss anything.

A holistic pediatrician may incorporate into his practice strategies such as nutrition, Chinese herbal medicine, homeopathy, massage, and aromatherapy and be open to listening to you and helping to support your choices.

Lamaze Technique

Lamaze focuses on *you* being in charge of your birth and gearing your birth around not using medications. Lamaze courses are typically about twelve hours long and cover labor positions, massage and relaxation techniques during birth, and some postpartum support such as breastfeeding. This isn't used so prevalently anymore, in favor of the Bradley Method below.

The Bradley Method

Like Lamaze, the Bradley Method also focuses on a nonmedicated approach and has an added emphasis on the partner as the primary birth coach. Although this method prepares you to give birth without medications, it also prepares you for the possibility of unexpected situations, such an as emergency cesarean section. You'll also get a chance in the Bradley Method to rehearse your birth.

Alexander Technique

The Alexander Technique focuses on body awareness elements such as movement, balance, and flexibility and can be practiced weekly during pregnancy. It aims to help you not only during pregnancy, but also during pushing and recovery after childbirth.

HypnoBirthing

Also called the Mongan Method, HypnoBirthing employs self-hypnosis techniques. It is usually a series of four to five classes with a lot of material that you can supplement via the Internet or guided visualization audios.

Where to Find Birthing Classes

To locate childbirth classes near you, ask your obstetrician, doula, midwife, or friends who have attended birth classes. There are also plenty of books and videos you can explore from home. See the resource section for a few books that I recommend on this topic.

At the end of the day, I don't recommend being overly focused on exactly what technique you'd like to use or exactly how you'd like your birth to go. It's wonderful to have intentions and education and to map out your idea for your birth plan, but also valuable to remain open to discovering what you actually need along the way and have the right people attending your birth to help guide these ideals and choices in a safe way. Honestly, I think that most of this type of attention and preparing should go toward the aftermath of birth. Birth tends to go how it goes, and you get through it. The postpartum period, however, can greatly benefit from planning and plotting your support systems. See birth plan section in month seven for more on this.

....

HOMEMADE HUMMUS

Hummus is made from chickpeas (garbanzo beans) and sesame butter, both rich in iron and calcium. This dip can be used as a nutritious spread on sprouted grain toast, crackers, or raw vegetables.

You can also combine hummus, brown rice, avocado, vegetables, and/or kelp noodles onto a sheet of nori (the nutrient-dense seaweed used to make sushi) and roll it up for a healthy snack.

Ingredients

> 2 cups cooked and drained or canned chickpeas
>
> ½ cup tahini (sesame butter)
>
> ¼ cup extra-virgin olive oil
>
> ½ teaspoon ground cumin
>
> ½ teaspoon paprika
>
> Juice of one lemon
>
> Salt and ground black pepper to taste
>
> Chopped fresh parsley for garnish

Directions

Blend everything except for the parsley until smooth (adjust salt and lemon as desired). Put in bowl and top with parsley.

....

Infant CPR

Infant CPR is important to know should you ever find yourself in a position to need it. Doing a course while still pregnant is probably more realistic than when you're a new mom, but if you don't get around to it, there are some great instructional courses online. Research has shown that videos can be as efficacious as in-person training. I highly recommend that any care provider you may enlist for your child is also certified.

Baby Shower

Most ancient cultures throughout history have some record of what we would now call a baby shower. Traditionally, these are events centered on the mother-to-be. Although the modern emphasis tends to shift this onto sprinkling the little-one-to-be with gifts, perhaps think of how to incorporate receiving some nurturing treats and attention for yourself during this time too.

The way you choose to care for yourself and the manner in which you welcome your newborn is not just about your child, but also an important element of your transition into motherhood. So, however you choose to celebrate with those around you, make sure you are at the center of the celebration—this may be one of the last times you revel in that feeling for a while.

Checklist for Month Four

- Investigate childbirth classes.
- Take an infant CPR course.
- Get a body pillow or other props to help with sleeping.
- Start or continue probiotics.

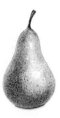

Month Five
Centering

- Baby is 10.5 inches and 12.7 ounces.
- He or she is producing meconium (a dark, tarry substance that's part of baby's first poop).
- If it's a girl, she already has roughly 6 million eggs in her ovaries.

- Baby is 11 inches and 16 ounces.
- He or she is now sleeping in cycles.

- Baby is still about 11 inches and 16 ounces. (They're entering one of first phases of relative dormancy, where they're conserving themselves before their next growth spurt. So, you'll notice during these times a few weeks here and there where they don't grow a ton.)
- The nipples are formed.
- Baby can hear the outside world.

- Baby is still about 11 inches and 16 ounces.

- Skin is becoming more opaque and pinkish (due to forming capillaries).
- This week marks the first time baby could potentially be viable outside the uterus.

....

East-West Fetal Development

In Chinese medicine, month five—the center of your pregnancy timeline—is also associated with the center or source of your energy, the Spleen. This Spleen system can be thought of like the mitochondria in the cells that produce adenosine triphosphate (ATP), or energy. Since food and nutrients are the source of energy, we can also equate the Spleen with the digestive system.

This month, your body is drawing on even more of your resources to support large growth spurts in baby. This is an important time to nourish yourself with easy-to-digest foods so that less of your resources are going to breaking down complex things and more are going to supporting the distribution of the nutrients to all of the places they need to go. When the Spleen gets taxed it gives out a little bit, and symptoms such as fatigue, swelling, hemorrhoids, gas, bloating, and muscle soreness can occur. So even though you may have more energy overall, keep resting as much as possible. It's the best remedy for keeping the Spleen strong and keeping you and baby energized and incubating.

Fibromyalgia

Fibromyalgia is a tender subject. There have been debates about this condition for as long as it has been named, but regardless of the origin of the discomfort—the mind or the body—the reality is an intermingling of symptoms that are perceivable to you, and now there are more standardized and accepted ways of distinguishing fibromyalgia from other conditions with similar presentations in order to arrive at an appropriate diagnosis.

Many women with fibromyalgia report that it gets progressively worse throughout pregnancy. This makes sense, since an already burdened musculoskeletal system only becomes more burdened with the increasing demands of carrying a baby. There are no consistent adverse outcomes of pregnancy or birth that are solely related to fibromyalgia, though. It's mostly about managing your comfort levels—physically and emotionally.

During pregnancy, you can approach the physical symptoms primarily as an inflammatory issue and incorporate foods from the Easy Anti-Inflammatory Eating Plan for Candida sidebar, and approach the emotional aspects through mindfulness techniques or other interventions that you've sought out to help you investigate and cope with this mess of sensations.

Chronic Fatigue Syndrome

Chronic fatigue syndrome (CFS) is a common co-condition with fibromyalgia and predominately affects women. Perhaps it evolved from carrying and raising children for millennia! A lot of women with CFS are intimidated about going through the process of pregnancy, which of course adds more components of fatigue and other physical stressors, and rightly so. Although women with CFS *do* get through their pregnancies, it's often not without difficulty.

If you are thinking of becoming pregnant, and you have CFS, this is a good time to evaluate your support network, because you might find that you need to rely on it more than usual. It's also important to note that postpartum depression is about three times higher in women with CFS. Preparing a solid support team is essential. Lining up some help beyond just your partner for when baby comes may give you some peace of mind and alleviate the extra exhaustion that comes with anticipating fatigue.

Of course, CFS doesn't have to just remain a resolute condition either. Utilizing some approaches such as acupuncture and staying on top of nutrition can help build stamina and health. Having a child is exhausting no matter how you cut it, or how you go into it, but paying attention to rest and different layers of support can help bolster as much energy as is available to you.

Maternal Phenylketonuria

Phenylketonuria (PKU) is caused by a mutation in a gene that helps create the enzyme needed to break down the amino acid phenylalanine. During pregnancy, abnormal levels of PKU can cross the placental barrier and cause intellectual disabilities, seizures, and other congenital issues in babies.

Both parents must pass along a copy of the mutated PKU gene in order for their child to develop the condition. Although babies born to mothers with high phenylalanine levels may have complications at birth, most don't actually inherit PKU and won't need to follow a PKU diet after birth. The heel stick test performed on newborns screens for this condition.

Maternal PKU is addressed through dietary management, which includes following a low-phenylalanine diet: avoid foods that are high in protein, such as milk, cheese, nuts, or meats; avoid NutraSweet (aspartame) since it contains phenylalanine; and limit fruits. You should also typically take a medical formula containing amino acids and other nutrients specific for regulating PKU.

Shortness of Breath

Breathe easy, because shortness of breath is normal when a baby is compressing your diaphragm. You're not necessarily out of shape; you're just pregnant, and your respiratory and cardiovascular systems are working harder. Utilizing breathing and mindfulness exercises during this time can be a way to counterbalance some of the anxiety that can result from shallow breathing, as well as help you deepen your breathing to whatever extent is available. Swimming is also a great way to build respiratory capacity. Any breath work during pregnancy helps to build your relationship to breathing and can ultimately contribute to your labor process.

Measles, Mumps, Rubella, and Chicken Pox

You are not a reservoir for infection during pregnancy, but you are a little more vulnerable to some infections—not just because you're pregnant, but also because there's a developing baby involved. So, the impact is potentially different. Contagious diseases such as measles, mumps, rubella, and chicken pox can pose serious health risks for the baby, but since pregnancy doesn't mix with the measles-mumps-rubella (MMR) or varicella (chicken pox) vaccines, give it your best shot to minimize the exposure to these infectious diseases.

Planning Maternity Leave

By this point in your pregnancy, your priorities may naturally be shifting, and stepping away from work or planning maternity leave may not seem as daunting or uncompelling as it may have originally. Yet as you're mapping out your maternity leave, you may be battling a feeling that you are abandoning other pursuits that you've worked hard to attain. There may be more options for your continued involvement or return to work than you think. You may also stand to be influenced by what still feels like a priority for you after baby arrives. Many women firmly plan on returning to work after two months, only to discover that even at six months it can feel too soon.

It's different for everyone, so I recommend exploring your options so that you're equipped with the tools to modify your leave as you go along. Most countries besides the United States give you a year, and from all the women I've seen, this is a pretty good standard. Also, don't forget about exploring your partner having some time off too.

Some practical strategies include reviewing your employee handbook and/or working with your HR department to learn about any coverage or benefits available to you. The Family and Medical Leave Act (FMA) states that if you work for a company that has at least fifty employees within a seventy-five-mile radius, and you've been there for a year, you are eligible for twelve paid weeks off. The National Conference of State Legislatures can be explored to learn about your individual state's policies about maternity leave.

Will and Guardian

It can be a challenging process to consider the end of your life while contemplating the beginning of a new one, but this legal protection may ensure that if anything unforeseen happens, your child always has the life you want for her, cared for by the people you want her to be cared for by.

If you don't already have a trusted lawyer, you can contact the American Bar Association for help in finding the right lawyer to execute this for you.

Enlarged Shoe Size

If the shoe fits . . . or more accurately, used to fit but doesn't anymore, this is due to all of the fluid changes and swelling in your lower body. Many women experience swelling in their feet and often have to start wearing a whole different shoe size while pregnant, and sometimes this becomes a new, permanent shoe size.

Glucose Screening and Glucose Tolerance Test (GTT)

Glucose screening is routinely done around week twenty-four to assess your blood sugar. The test involves downing a glucose solution and waiting around the lab for an hour, then having blood drawn to determine how efficiently your body is processing sugar.

Bear in mind, a positive test doesn't necessarily indicate gestational diabetes, and if the levels are high, you'll come back in for a more intense three-hour glucose tolerance test (GTT). Be sure not to eat for at least two hours before the first screening, and a longer fast for the GTT. Both of these tests can make you feel sick. So, bring snacks for afterward.

See gestational diabetes section for more details.

Linea Nigra

Are you ready to draw the line with pregnancy symptoms? Well, it's already drawn for you—on your abdomen, where the abdominal muscles start to separate to allow pregnancy growth. As you continually interface with the changes in your body during pregnancy, you'll find that some are abstract and internal, and some are outwardly visible. One of these visual markers of your pregnancy might be the darkening of a line that extends from your pubic bone to your belly button. This line is called the *linea nigra* and is pigmentation that has been linked to changes in sex hormones, such as estrogen, a dominant hormone in pregnancy.

In case you're not a fan of linea nigra, it often fades after pregnancy.

Hemorrhoids

Hemorrhoids are not always visible, but you can tell they are around when you start feeling itchy and raw and perhaps notice bright red spotting or bleeding during bowel movements. It's a good idea to check with your practitioner to rule out any other causes of bleeding, but once you're confident that you are experiencing these uncomfortable markers of pregnancy, read on.

Hemorrhoids happen when impaired blood circulation (going more to baby than your intestines and limbs) leads to accumulation in the blood vessels of your rectum. Further inflammation occurs with abrasion to this delicate tissue due to straining from constipation and the unavoidable pressure on the lower abdominal organs from pregnancy. Your body is going through a lot, and hemorrhoids are a literal sort of "giving out," but don't give up.

In Chinese medicine, hemorrhoids are caused by a sinking in the Spleen system. Sort of like the Western idea of prolapse. To give this system, and hopefully your hemorrhoids, a lift, you can target your digestion by eating easy-to-process foods. This will help the whole digestive tract from start to finish. Eating enough protein helps promote proper fluid exchange in the body, and good proteins can also minimize unnecessary swelling. Sweet potatoes provide a good fix for fiber, and also happen to work very specifically towards boosting this Spleen system.

Other foods that can assist you in sorting through this uncomfortable time by being easy to digest and further supporting the Spleen system include adzuki beans, apples, lamb or beef (especially stewed), black beans, carrots, cherries, cinnamon, dates, eggplant, ginger, grapes, halibut, mackerel, nutmeg, oats, peas, raspberries, rutabaga, sauerkraut, spelt, squash, turnips, and yogurt with live cultures.

It was postulated that enhanced levels of vitamin C in Captain Robert Falcon Scott's rations during his 1910 expedition to the Antarctic may have significantly improved his survival chances. Since the symptoms of pregnancy can feel like your own arduous expedition through uncharted lands, we can at least draw on our modern knowledge to improve survival, and also well-being. Ascorbic acid, or vitamin C, may help reduce damage to the digestive tract by astringing and decreasing bleeding. Some foods that aren't citrusy or spicy (which can exacerbate heartburn), but *are* high in vitamin C,

....

SITZ BATH FOR HEMORRHOIDS

Preparing the herbs:

Put a small handful each of calendula flowers, comfrey leaves, rosemary, and sage leaves* into a large, nonreactive kitchen pot and pour 10 cups of hot (not boiling) water over your bouquet.

Let this cool to room temperature (may take several hours, or you can let it sit overnight). Strain into a jar and keep in fridge for multiple uses.

* See the resources section for where to order dried herbs.

Preparing the sitz bath:

You can get a plastic basin from a drugstore or medical supply store that fits over your toilet (get some reading material too, since you'll be soaking for awhile). Warm up equal proportions of your herb mixture with plain warm or cold water to appropriately fill your basin (experiment to find a temperature that works best).

Add 1 cup Epsom salts

Add 1 tablespoon witch hazel

Soak for 15 to 20 minutes

For a simple version of the above, you can add a handful of black tea to a partially filled warm bathtub and soak for the same amount of time.

Finish with a topical swipe of a fresh aloe vera leaf (split it open to reveal the salve inside) or bottled, pure aloe vera gel (make sure it doesn't have an alcohol base or paraben preservatives).

....

PUMPKIN SOUP FOR YOU
AND YOUR LITTLE PUMPKIN

1 small pumpkin (can substitute 2 cans organic pumpkin purée)

1 tablespoon coconut oil

1 yellow onion, finely chopped

¼ teaspoon dried sage

¼ cup pumpkin seeds, toasted

Plain yogurt with live cultures

Directions

Bake whole pumpkin at 350 degrees Fahrenheit until soft (approximately forty minutes). Remove from oven, cut open, and remove seeds. Scoop pumpkin meat into a bowl. Heat up deep-sided pan with 1 tablespoon coconut oil. Add onion and sauté until onions soften and turn slightly and golden. Add sage, cook for three more minutes and add pumpkin meat. Stir for five minutes over heat to incorporate flavors. Transfer to blender with 2 cups stock (see Boosted-Up Chicken Stock recipe on page 46). Add up to one more cup of stock until you reach your desired consistency.

Top with toasted pumpkin seeds and a dollop of fresh yogurt.

....

include dried currants and parsley. If your stomach can tolerate citrus, try the Soothing Thyme and Honey Digestif recipe on page 94.

One last note on treating hemorrhoids: you can use herbs to topically soothe and astringe. An easy, nonmessy way to do this is with a sitz bath, which is great to get the supplies for anyway since you'll really want to use a Sitz Bath after birth! (See recipe.)

Gas and Bloating

Bloating and gas come from the same pregnancy origins, also related to the Spleen system "giving out." Bloating (distention) is the preamble to gas, but where bloating may be physically uncomfortable, gas can cause both physical and social discomfort. The main reason for these symptoms early on in pregnancy is that there's an extra amount of progesterone being produced. This is the "sluggish hormone" (think back to PMS). Later on in pregnancy, as your uterus grows even bigger, your intestines become compressed, which slows your digestion and contributes to accumulation. To top it off, some pregnancy hormones have muscle-relaxing effects (comes in handy for birth, but not so much right now) that make it even harder for you to control your flatulence.

SPLEEN-BOOSTING ACORN SQUASH STUFFED WITH LAMB AND CINNAMON

Ingredients

1 tablespoon coconut oil

1 large carrot, shredded

1 shallot, minced

1 fennel bulb, finely chopped

1 acorn squash

4 ounces ground lamb (beef will work too)

1 egg, whisked

2 teaspoons cinnamon

½ teaspoon nutmeg

½ teaspoon sea salt

½ teaspoon pepper

Directions

Preheat oven to 350 degrees Fahrenheit. Using a sharp knife, cut the acorn squash in half, lengthwise, from stem to end. Use a spoon to scoop out the seeds and stringy stuff in the center of each half and discard it. Place each half in a casserole dish, cut side down. Add about a ¼-inch of water to the bottom of the baking pan and bake for about twenty minutes until squash is soft but not too mushy. In a pan, sauté shallot, shredded carrots, and fennel in coconut oil. Once the vegetables are soft, put them in a mixing bowl with the meat, egg, and spices. Mix thoroughly with clean hands. Fill each acorn squash half with filling. Dump the water out of the casserole dish and bake for twenty more minutes, face up, until meat is thoroughly cooked.

To counterbalance gas and bloating, try to identify which foods your digestion might not like. The primary culprits that usually cause gas have components that make them a little less digestible:

- carbohydrates
- dairy
- fizzy sodas
- foods that have substantial soluble fibers—peas and beans
- vegetables—artichokes, asparagus, Brussels sprouts, broccoli, cabbage, onions—that contain raffinose sugar (which is technically indigestible to humans)

Exercise also helps healthy peristalsis (the muscle contractions that help your digestive system process food). So, eat small meals and keep moving—both your body and bowels.

TIP: Digestive enzymes can help with gas and bloating. A pregnancy-safe way to incorporate digestive enzymes is to eat small portions of sauerkraut or miso soup with each meal. This helps break down the gases in your breaking-down digestive system.

Checklist for Month Five

- Schedule your glucose tolerance test and longer glucose screening if necessary.
- Look into preparing will and guardianship documents.
- Continue planning maternity leave.

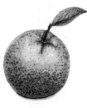

Month Six

Ripening

WEEK TWENTY-FIVE

- Baby is 14 inches and 2 pounds.

WEEK TWENTY-SIX

- Baby is remaining about 14 inches and 2 pounds.
- Baby's eyes are developing and will open soon.
- He or she continues to practice breathing by taking gulps of amniotic fluid.

WEEK TWENTY-SEVEN

- Baby is holding strong around 14 inches and 2 pounds.
- Lungs are rapidly developing.

WEEK TWENTY-EIGHT

- At the start of your third trimester, baby's growth remains on par with the last couple of weeks.
- Lungs are fully matured.
- Baby can smell what you're smelling.
- You can start doing "kick counts" this week (see page 147).

East-West Fetal Development

In Chinese medicine, month six is governed by the Stomach system. The Stomach is paired with the digestive functions of the Spleen that we explored in month five. Where the Spleen is more about what you're taking in, the Stomach breaks down and uses that material for fuel. From an Eastern and Western point of view, when the Stomach isn't adequately processing, it rebels and creates symptoms such as acid regurgitation (reflux) and hiccups.

Let's also remember that baby is starting to physically compress the stomach now. So, there is some inevitable revolt. The best strategy is to eat frequent small meals from here on out and minimize dry, dehydrated foods like crackers, popcorn, and dried fruit, which can leach the moisture out of the stomach and intestines, contributing to constipation, or spicy foods, which can agitate the lining of the stomach and intestines even more.

Third Trimester Checkup

Your six-month checkup will monitor baby's growth and position and look at the amount of amniotic fluid and the position of the placenta.

Body Art

Fifty percent of body ornamentation is done on women these days. Preexisting tattoos and piercings, besides potentially becoming distorted if they're in an area that is growing and stretching, for the most part don't interfere with pregnancy. Some exceptions are that nipple piercings can impair breastfeeding, and in an emergency, oral piercings may interfere with managing opening an airway. I recommend taking your jewelry out during this period to be extra safe.

There is also some very loose debate about introducing tattoo pigments into other areas of the body during an epidural (this is only relevant for low-back tattoos) and creating the potential for some subsequent health problems, but again, this is a very controversial idea. However, knowing that there's a potential risk might factor into your decision-making process about having an epidural.

Third Trimester Vaccine Considerations

A current recommendation by the Center for Disease Control (CDC) and American College of Obstetricians and Gynecologists (ACOG) is to get a diphtheria, tetanus, and pertussis (DTaP) vaccine during your third trimester, with the idea that it passes along passive immunity to your newborn. They are usually administered between twenty-seven and thirty-six weeks, because they take a couple of weeks to kick in.

It is worth noting that the CDC states "the benefits of vaccinating pregnant women usually outweigh potential risks when the likelihood of disease exposure is high, when infection would pose a risk to the mother or fetus, and when the vaccine is unlikely to cause harm, but the effectiveness of maternal antibodies in preventing infant pertussis is not yet known." You can factor this in to your ongoing exploration of your choices around vaccines and continued exploration of the risk-to-benefit ratio. Alongside considering your own circumstances, incorporating information from your healthcare providers can help you arrive at your best decision.

Vascular Changes

Vascular (circulation) changes are normal during pregnancy because of the upped estrogen levels and increased blood volume, which can cause expansion and congestion of your blood vessels.

Spider veins can appear on your face, neck, and arms. Varicose derives from the Latin *varix*, which means "twisted," and these bulging veins can twist along throughout your body both in visible areas as well as on your vulva or present as rectal hemorrhoids. This type of bulging comes from the same mechanism that causes other types of fluid leakage during pregnancy, such as edema (swelling) in your face, eyelids, and extremities. These blood flow issues can also cause flushing in your face, changes in your body temperature, and a generally marbled look. Support stockings and pregnancy belts, along with consistent, moderate exercise, are the main ways to support your vascular system at this stage.

Bleeding Gums

Many women complain of sensitive gums that are more prone to bleeding during pregnancy. A rise in hormones can alter your body's response to normal bacteria and predispose you to inflammation or periodontal infections even to the point of potentially causing benign tumors on your gums. Obvious prevention through brushing, flossing, and regular dental checkups is essential for maintaining oral health. Make sure your dentist is up to date on appropriate pregnancy-safe dental hygiene.

Bleeding gums may also be indicative of preeclampsia. So, be sure to check in with your healthcare provider about that.

Leg Cramps

Many women experience leg cramps in the second half of pregnancy. This can be from increasing weight placing demands on your muscles, and if your level of exercise has slowed a bit and you're recovering from the carbohydrate intake of the first trimester, there may also be a buildup of lactic and pyruvic acids, which are by-products of sugar and starch, and get more concentrated when there's less blood flow in the legs.

The solution is to *move*. Walk (with comfy, supportive shoes), swim, stretch, and wiggle your toes at any given opportunity. At the same time, stay hydrated with electrolytes and boost up on calcium-rich foods (found in month one) and magnesium sources such as the Morning Mocktail recipe (page 27).

As ever, we return to the science behind the folklore. The old "I'm pregnant and craving pickles" thing might just indicate another iteration of a pregnant woman knowing exactly what she needs. An easy way to get electrolytes and magnesium in is through pickle juice, which has been shown to help relieve muscle cramps. Professional athletes use this remedy for endurance—and let's face it, pregnancy is an endurance exercise.

NOTE: If leg cramps are a constant versus occasional pain, check in with your practitioner to rule out a blood clot.

....

IN A PICKLE WITH CRAMPS?

This pickle juice cocktail works wonders to replenish you. About an hour before bedtime, dilute half a glass (about 4 ounces) of pickle juice with half a glass of water and drink. This timing targets when cramps are most likely to strike (during sleep) but leaves you time for a bathroom stop before bed.

For another good cramp remedy, see the recipe for the Electrolyte Refresher in month one.

....

ESSENTIAL OIL MOUTHWASH FOR SWOLLEN GUMS

Myrrh is a traditional herb that used to be as valuable as gold, and it will probably be held in equally high esteem by you when use it as a mouthwash. Some of myrrh's active ingredients are antimicrobial, antiseptic, and anti-inflammatory and contribute to reducing infection and pain in your sore gums when used topically. In fact, Greek soldiers used to apply myrrh oil to wounds to stop the bleeding.

You can make an easy and effective anti-inflammatory mouthwash by mixing together two drops of myrrh essential oil with a cup of warm water and using it as a daily rinse.

....

DAILY SALTWATER RINSE

There's an ocean of things to deal with in pregnancy, and you can add the discomfort in your gums to this list, in the second trimester in particular. Let the sea soothe you with this easy saline mouthwash:

Pour one teaspoon of good quality sea salt into a cup of warm water and swish and spit before bed.

....

What to Pack for the Hospital

If you're planning to give birth in the hospital, here's a short list of what you should pack. The main thing to remember is to travel light. You'll be bringing more home than you came with. Once labor begins, most women don't use many props, and if you imagined you'd be interspersing contractions with meandering activities, I'd advise that even if you have the wherewithal for that, use your in-between times to really rest:

- A change of clothes, including underwear and comforting items such as slippers and a robe
- Something to read or watch in case you stay at the hospital during very early labor
- A hair band, if your hair is long enough to pull back off your face
- Toiletries
- A camera
- A large exercise ball (great for sitting on or draping over during labor)
- Blanket and warm baby clothes (including hat) for taking baby home
- Diapers if you have a special preference. Otherwise, the hospital will give you some
- Some hearty food for after the birth—either bring or enlist someone to bring for you
- Make sure to have your car seat installed in advance so you don't have to struggle with it at the hospital.

While you're undergoing a hospital birth, you can't eat or drink, so don't bother to bring snacks. The rationale for this is that you may need anesthesia during birth interventions, but, ironically, a nonhydrated, low-blood-sugar laboring woman is less likely to muster the stamina for a full birth process and so potentially will need that very intervention. It may be worth discussing with your physician that there was a large study of over 3,000 women that concluded women should be free to eat and drink what they please during labor to see if there's any wiggle room to snack as needed.

Restless Leg Syndrome

Restless leg syndrome (RLS) has been shown to be associated with a number of complications in pregnancy such as preeclampsia and increased rates of C-sections. Some thoughts around the contributors to RLS are low iron and ferritin levels, and vitamin D and calcium deficiency. So, boost up on foods rich in these, and supplement if needed.

Anemia

Is your healthy glow of pregnancy fading—or have you even experienced one yet? You might not just be experiencing the normal lack of verve that can come with being in the late stages of pregnancy. You might actually have anemia. It can be difficult to tease out the symptoms of anemia from normal pregnancy symptoms, but be alert for feeling not only fatigued, but also weak and dizzy. Other anemia symptoms can include headaches, shortness of breath, irritability, heart palpitations, restless leg syndrome, running colder than usual, and paleness.

Incidentally, the concept of vampires came from a real disease called *porphyria* and its associated cravings—characterized in part by anemia. Before we had good diagnostic sense, these anemic folks who looked very pale and craved blood were monsterized. However, we can learn from this history. Food cravings are often indicative of what we need, like bloody, red meat for anemia. Sometimes, though, our bodies guide us astray in an attempt to get certain nutrients. For instance, pica is the craving for nonfoods like paper, clay, sand, paint, or ice in an effort to get appropriate nutrients. So, do check your cravings against the list on pages 42–44 of actual iron-rich and blood-building foods.

It's important to treat anemia in pregnancy, and the first place to turn is iron. Iron is present in every cell in the body and is essential for the production of hemoglobin, which is the protein in red blood cells that carries oxygen. During pregnancy, you have 50 percent more blood (by volume) than normal, so naturally you require more iron to make more hemoglobin to support that additional circulation and nourish the needs of the placenta and baby. Additionally, proper iron can minimize the potential of preterm birth, decrease risk of needing a blood transfusion after birth, and has been linked to an aspect of offsetting postpartum depression.

Iron deficiency is a less severe gradient of iron-deficient anemia. The highest iron demands actually happen during the third trimester, when requirements for absorbed iron increase, and if you enter into actual anemia (hemoglobin measures less than 110 g/L in the first and third trimester and less than 105 g/L in the second trimester), or if your ferritin (a protein in the cells that stores iron) is less than 30 microg/l, you should consider supplementation of 80 to 100 mg of ferrous iron per day. (You can halve that dose if your ferritin is 30 to 70 microg/l.)

As a more general guideline, supplementing with 40 mg ferrous iron per day from eighteen weeks on appears to adequately prevent iron deficiency and iron deficiency anemia in most women, not only during pregnancy but also postpartum, and, of course, focus on getting iron from food sources.

To maximize iron absorption, take iron pills on an empty stomach with water or orange juice (the vitamin C helps with absorption). Avoid taking them with milk, because calcium interferes with absorption. Other hinderers include coffee and tea.

ALWAYS KEEP IRON PILLS AWAY FROM CHILDREN THAT MIGHT ALREADY BE IN YOUR HOUSEHOLD. A SINGLE ADULT DOSE CAN BE POISONOUS FOR A SMALL CHILD.

When you are iron deficient, your gut is already primed for higher iron absorption. Iron supplementation, however, can lead to constipation. In an attempt to not compound the issue, check out the constipation section (pages 88–91) for how to offset some of the unwanted side effects of iron supplementation.

Sickle Cell Disease

Sickle cell disease (SCD) is the most common inherited disease worldwide. It can lead to numerous health problems, but is most readily associated with anemia and intermittent, severe pain. It also happens to be a secondary protection against malaria (many people with SCD happen to inhabit malaria-infested areas), which can remind us that many things that seem dire may have hidden benefits, but of course this is a serious disease in and of itself,

Iron-Rich Foods

Pregnancy-friendly, iron-rich foods that you can't eat enough of include apricots (fresh and dried), beans (especially butter beans and lima beans), beef, beets, blackstrap molasses, broccoli, chicken, dates, figs, lentils, leafy greens, oatmeal, potatoes (with the skin on), prunes, pumpkin seeds, raisins, salmon, sardines in oil, sesame seeds, spinach, tofu, turkey, wheat germ, and whole grain breads.

and even more so in pregnancy. Pregnant women with SCD should seek out a multidisciplinary team with experience in high-risk pregnancies and receive regular monitoring for preeclampsia and fetal growth changes.

Hypertension (High Blood Pressure), Preeclampsia, and Edema

During early pregnancy, the heart works about 50 percent harder to supply important organs such as the uterus with more blood flow. The pressure your uterus puts on the blood vessels that return blood from your legs to your heart and the pressure on the nerves in your lower body result in blood flow and fluid changes. This pressure apexes around sixteen to twenty weeks into pregnancy, and can present as hypertension (high blood pressure) and/or edema—fluid accumulating under the surface of your legs, which makes them appear swollen.

During pregnancy, there is also an increased retention of sodium (salt), which leads to even more fluid retention. These things together can create the ever-so-sought-after cankles. High blood pressure (defined as 140/90 or more) can have some notable repercussions. It's important to talk to your medical practitioner if you are suffering from it.

Edema in the lower body without a rise in blood pressure is not dangerous, but it can cause symptoms such as pain, feelings of heaviness, cramps (especially at night), and pins and needles. When edema is present in conjunction with raised blood pressure, it's important to look out for preeclampsia.

The kidneys are also an integral part of the physiology of blood pressure changes, and changes in kidney function during pregnancy can contribute to some of the blood pressure complications. But, when the heart and kidneys are both working overtime, preeclampsia is even more of a risk.

If you have a pre-existing kidney disease, this adds into the mix, on top of the normal, pregnancy-related enhanced kidney function that's normal. Although this poses a potential risk for preeclampsia, many women experience a temporary resolve in their underlying or pre-existing conditions while pregnant. Other risk factors for preeclampsia include diabetes mellitus, thrombophilia, pre-existing hypertension, a first-degree relative who's had preeclampsia, a father who was born from a pregnancy complicated by preeclampsia, or low vitamin C levels. If you have increased risk factors, these can be hints to start to preemptively manage and closely monitor any warning signs.

It's normal for blood volume and pressure changes to occur and for the heart to work a little harder during pregnancy, but true hypertension happens in one out of every ten pregnancies. The typical signs of preeclampsia are a rapid rise in blood pressure along with protein in the urine (although not every woman exhibits these symptoms). Additional tests may reveal an elevation of uric acid in the urine and a decrease in the glomerular filtration rate, which speak to how hard the kidneys are working.

There are several reasons to be wary if you are at risk for preeclampsia. Short-term complications include risk of preterm delivery, cesarean section, placental abruption, central nervous system (CNS) injuries such as seizures (eclampsia), strokes, kidney damage, and liver damage—including HELLP syndrome (hemolysis, elevated liver enzymes, and low platelets). Sometimes the above can result in fetal growth restriction or respiratory difficulties in baby. Having said all of this, multiple studies have shown that preeclampsia may have some protective effects against mothers developing malignant cancers. So, nature may have some wisdom if you're facing preeclampsia.

In addition to working with your physician to determine if you need management with medication (generally diuretics, which, although they are typically considered safe for breastfeeding, can decrease milk production; so take that into account if you're having any trouble with breast feeding), close monitoring of you and baby to determine the earliest time to safely induce delivery may be an appropriate solution. The delivery of the baby (and of

---

Relaxin

Relaxin is a hormone that is secreted during pregnancy and plays a role in helping to widen the blood vessels to accommodate the increased flow and pressure. Keeping an eye out for low relaxin levels in the first trimester may be a helpful indicator for increased potential for developing preeclampsia later in pregnancy.

---

course the placenta) usually helps preeclampsia begin to resolve and minimizes potential threats to you or baby.

Babymoon

A honeymoon was originally called such because newly married couples were given enough mead (honey wine) to get them intoxicated enough to discover nuptial bliss, but pregnancy is a far more sobering experience, and a little pre-baby jaunt may be just the recipe to restore some adventure and intimacy. I don't necessarily recommend flying while pregnant (see travel section), so think about planning a pleasant and relaxing road trip, or even plan a staycation in your home or area.

I'm of the school that life doesn't stop when you have a baby. So, I don't think of the babymoon as the last vestige of your freedom, but life certainly will change. As you ready yourself for the next stage, consider planning a treat for you and yours to focus on each other and set the precedent of your existing relationship being the primary relationship—even after baby. After all, this is the foundation that burgeoned a baby in the first place.

Pregnancy-Related Skin Conditions

Here's the skinny on your skin: As blood flow increases during this trimester to accommodate the growing metabolic needs of your baby, you'll experience increased blood flow to organs such as your kidneys. This brings more blood to your vessels, which also increases oil-gland secretion. Along with increases in androgen levels (thought of as a male hormone, but present in both men and women), this can lead to development or worsening of acne. From a Chinese medicine perspective, skin conditions often involve the blood in a different way: "excess" (generated from things such as too many spicy foods) or "deficiency" (which can correlate to or be ebbing toward anemia—boost up on iron-rich foods for this). The point is that most skin conditions have a dietary relationship, which is a great first-line approach during pregnancy anyway.

Skin conditions during pregnancy have a few basic categories:

1. Something you already had that changes during pregnancy

2. Something hormone related

3. Something unique to pregnancy

If you have a known skin issue such as eczema or psoriasis, it can change during pregnancy—usually for the better. On the flip side, other splotches and blotches can arise during pregnancy. Fear not—most of these things spontaneously resolve after birth. In the meantime, you can always check in with your dermatologist.

Stretch Marks

You may be on the home stretch, yet only thinking about your stretch marks. Stretch marks, which usually look like pink or purple bands on areas where your body is growing to accommodate baby, occur in up to 90 percent of pregnant women by the third trimester. They are caused by the literal stretching of the skin, amplified by the effects of hormones such as relaxin that affect the skin's elastic fibers.

Stretch marks are mostly an issue of genetics—you either will or won't get them. But since they can be itchy, there are some strategies for tending to them. You can take a warm (not hot) bath with a couple of cups of very finely ground oatmeal or make (or buy) a soothing salve to apply. By the way, gotu kola has been studied for its effect in successfully preventing stretch marks. So, look for a cream that contains this plant, or blend up a homemade concoction using its extract (see Stretch Mark Oil recipe).

....

HONEY MASK WITH NUTMEG

Here's a basic at-home topical treatment for soothing blemishes or irritations.

Take a palmful of honey, which is antibacterial and moisture rich, and a pinch of nutmeg, which acts as an exfoliant, and rub them together. Apply to your face, neck, chest, or just about anywhere you're breaking out. Let the mask sit for ten to fifteen minutes. Wash away with warm water.

The honey will drip right off—no sticking, only a healthy glow!

....

OATMEAL BATH FOR ITCHY SKIN

Put one cup of oatmeal into a coffee filter or a muslin bag and tie it shut with a rubber band or string. Toss it into the bath as you fill the tub up with tepid (never hot, while pregnant) water, and when full, you can add an optional cup of buttermilk. Soak in your sanctuary for at least ten minutes.

....

Eczema and Psoriasis

A Turkish physician from the 1400s recommended acupuncture for eczema in his canonical medical text, and modern research would support this finding—acupuncture has been compared to antihistamines for its equivalent effect to relieve itching, which in a deeper sense means addressing the root of the inflammation that's presenting topically.

And as mentioned before, anti-inflammatory dietary strategies are the first course of action for these persistent and unseemly skin flares (see the Easy Anti-Inflammatory Eating Plan for Candida sidebar for food and eating suggestions).

Hyper-Pigmentation

Nearly all women experience some pigment changes during pregnancy, mostly around the areolae or armpits. Scars and moles can darken too. At a certain stage, you really can't mask a pregnancy, especially since 70 percent

....

STRETCH MARK OIL
(Makes about one cup of oil)

Ingredients

⅓ cup almond, apricot, or jojoba oil (or a combination of all of them)

¼ cup macerated oil such as calendula or rose oil (you can make this in advance by soaking dried calendula flowers and/or rose petals in one of the above carrier oils for two weeks, then straining out the solids)

3 tablespoons avocado and/or hempseed oil

1 tablespoon evening primrose oil

1 teaspoon vitamin E oil

30 drops pregnancy-safe essential oil such as mandarin or ylang ylang

15 drops alcohol-free gotu kola extract (essential for its role in diminishing stretchmarks)

Mix all ingredients together and bottle, then rub-a-dub-dub onto your belly and breasts daily. Store in the fridge between uses.

Another down-and-dirty stretch mark solution is to simply use cocoa butter.

....

of women experience melasma, or "mask of pregnancy." It appears as a brownish or yellowish coloration on the face, kind of like a semipermanent decoration for a masquerade ball. Staying out of the sun can lessen the detriment. As with most changes in pregnancy, these pigmentation issues usually resolve postpartum.

Itching

Itching is a common skin irritation during pregnancy. Usually it's just annoying, but sometimes it can indicate intrahepatic cholestasis of pregnancy (ICP) or jaundice of pregnancy. With this, the itching is usually the

Did You Know That Your Baby's Cells Can Migrate to Your Skin During Pregnancy?

The abdominal rash known as polymorphic eruptions of pregnancy (PEP), previously known as PUPPP, is the most common pregnancy-specific skin situation, which usually involve the appearance of skin lesions after week thirty-four. It happens in about one out of three pregnancies, usually in the third trimester. We don't know why it happens, but PEP most likely involves the interaction between your and baby's immune systems. There's really nothing to do about it, but know that it usually goes away about three weeks after birth.

most intense on the palms of the hands and the soles of the feet, but it can be also unwieldy on the abdomen and other parts of the body.

ICP can cause vitamin K deficiency, which can lead to blood-clotting issues. If you have gallstones or a family history of gallstones, look out for ICP. Its presence during pregnancy can be associated with a higher risk of premature delivery. So if you're inordinately itchy, find out what's going on by investigating with your healthcare provider.

Impetigo Herpetiformis

Impetigo herpetiformis is a rare skin disorder that can appear during the second half of pregnancy. Whether this disorder is specific to pregnancy or is simply exacerbated by it is controversial. In addition to the pus-filled bumps (usually on the thighs, inner groin, and extremities), signs and symptoms of impetigo herpetiformis can include nausea, vomiting, diarrhea, fever, chills, and enlarged lymph nodes, usually without itching.

Western treatment for impetigo herpetiformis usually involves corticosteroids and antibiotics. Of course, your healthcare provider and/or dermatologist will help you properly differentiate what's going on and develop a course of action from there.

Lyme Disease

Pregnant or not pregnant, having Lyme disease, a bacterial infection, is a complicated matter. If you've been in an area with woodland creatures—especially if you know you've had a tick bite and you have symptoms such as persistent fatigue, joint aches, headaches, and/or a rash that looks like a bull's eye, Lyme disease is definitely something to rule out. But as Lyme disease also has a host of nonspecific symptoms, such as fatigue, which can be easily rolled into the pregnancy presentation, it can be hard to diagnose, and treatment strategies vary. Doxycylin is the first antibiotic of choice in Western medicine, but it can't be used in pregnancy because of the risks to the baby, including permanent discoloration of teeth and a possible impact on bone formation. So, you'll need to work with your team on looking at other antibiotics and treatment options.

There has been some great evidence that using a comprehensive herb and supplement regime as an effective approach for targeting Lyme disease. If the tick is still on you, lemon eucalyptus extract inhibits the tick from binding to the skin. Herbal therapy and supplements can continue to act on symptoms from an infection through the enhancement of natural killer-cell activity, which fights infection (antioxidants, astragalus, and mushroom b-glucan), inhibition of proinflammatory cytokine production with antioxidants (turmeric, EPA/DHA—basically fish oil—and boswellia), inactivation of the fibrinolytic system (COQ-10 and vitamin E), inhibition of tight junction degradation (vitamin D and N-acetylcysteine), and repair of the blood brain barrier (vitamin D and ginkgo biloba).

Human Immunodeficiency Virus (HIV) and Pregnancy

HIV can be a daunting diagnosis in general, and especially as an expecting mother, but there are many efficacious methods and medications available for reducing mother-to-child transmission.

While being HIV positive does not preclude having a healthy baby, there are some things you should do to help prevent passing the virus on. In most instances, HIV doesn't cross the placenta. So, the likely modes of transmission happen during birth and breastfeeding. C-sections have been shown to reduce baby's exposure, and if you opt for a vaginal delivery, avoiding an episiotomy (which increases the baby's potential exposure to blood) may help minimize risk as well. Although, bear in mind you may likely tear involuntarily. Most evidence points to limiting breastfeeding to six months, depending on your individual health status, or opting out of breastfeeding altogether.

HIV is not particularly different than many health concerns during pregnancy in that, alongside any appropriate medication, managing your nutrition is the optimal route for bolstering your and baby's immunity. Additionally, if you're not going to breastfeed, but are concerned about your baby getting the best possible nutrients, you have some relatively good options for high-quality formula these days and ways to enhance formula. See resource section for a formula recommendation.

Kick Counts

Starting around week twenty-eight, you may want to begin counting the number of kicks and other types of movement you feel from baby. This is an easy and noninvasive way to connect with and check on your baby.

You may notice that your baby is the most active after you eat or after exercise—these are good times to monitor the kicking. Lie on your left side to increase circulation and allow baby a full breadth of activity. According to American Congress of Obstetricians and Gynecologists (ACOG), you should feel at least ten movements (kicks, flutters, rolls, etc.) within a two-hour period. Look out for any deviations in your baby's normal routine.

If you notice a significant change, especially over a period of a few days, and after trying to kick start the kick counts with a good-sized meal and ice water to spark baby, check in with your healthcare provider.

Fetal Hiccups

It is a hiccup in your pregnancy, so to speak, but not a worrisome one. Fetal hiccups usually feel like a muscle twitch and are basically the baby practicing reflexes to prepare for activities such as eating and breathing. You can approach them much the same way as you do kick counts to monitor your baby's normal movement, which is the best gauge when assessing "normal."

Checklist for Month Six

- You can preregister at the hospital to avoid paperwork upon your arrival. This includes if you are intending to have a home birth and may need to be transported to the hospital.
- Identify a birth and/or postpartum doula if you're opting for this support.
- Start doing kick counts.
- Pick up items from the "What to Pack for the Hospital" checklist on page 136.

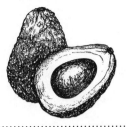

Month Seven
Processing

- Baby is 16 inches and 3 pounds.
- Fatty layer under skin continues to build.
- Buds for permanent teeth are forming in the gums.

- Baby is 16 inches and 3 pounds.
- Brain is now developing indentations, to accommodate important brain tissue and developments.
- Lanugo, the soft hair that has been covering baby, is starting to disappear. (The baby will end up swallowing it before birth, and it becomes part of their first poop!)
- Baby's bone marrow is taking over red-blood-cell production from the spleen.

- Baby is staying around last week's size and weight.
- All five senses are working and processing stimuli—such as reactions to light.
- Rapid brain growth continues to occur.

....

WEEK THIRTY-TWO

- Baby is still comfortable around 16 inches and 3 pounds.
- Many babies assume the head-down (labor-ready) position by this week.

....

East-West Fetal Development

Breathe deeply. Okay, more realistically: shallowly but frequently. This is the month of the Chinese Lung. The Lung system, includes our whole respiratory tract as well as our skin—our first two interfaces and boundaries against invading pathogens.

Just as keeping your immune system well is a priority in pregnancy, so is creating boundaries that enable you to focus on your task at hand and not overextend yourself. And just as breathing brings oxygen-rich regeneration to your cells, the Lung system is about renewal, so as you breathe in and breathe out, this is a great time to practice receiving and letting go—asking for help and disregarding the tasks you can't get to. It's great practice for impending motherhood.

The cyclical, involuntary nature of breathing is also a great thing to observe at this time. A guided, mindful, breath-orientated practice may help you move toward receptivity—especially during labor, when breath will truly be your guide.

Asthma

Asthma is one of the most common complications during pregnancy, and about a third of women with asthma find that it gets worse during pregnancy. Asthma can increase the risk of preeclampsia and preterm delivery, so it's important to manage it as well as you can and also keep monitoring your symptoms with your healthcare providers. As ever, nature is onto this issue, and the placenta releases substances that can help to mediate asthma.

Asthmatic spasms in your lungs can result from overstimulation of your parasympathetic nervous system. Stress reduction techniques (physical and emotional) can help you breathe a little easier. Additionally, a Mediterranean diet has shown protective effects on childhood asthma. So, to help prevent asthma in your newborn and keep yourself well nourished along the way, keep relying on good eating habits, including regular meals balanced with good protein, healthy sources of fats and oils, and lots of veggies. And be sure to boost up on antioxidants to help reduce the inflammation that comes with asthma. Magnesium has also shown bronchodilating (lung relaxing) effects. Add that to your regimen too.

Cystic Fibrosis

Cystic fibrosis transmembrane conductance regulator (CFTR) functions as a channel that regulates the transport of ions and the movement of water across the lining of your respiratory tract. Mutations in CFTR affect this innate immune function in the lung and result in exaggerated and ineffective inflammation in your airway that creates a buildup of mucus and also fails to push out pathogens. This clogging can lead to blockage, not only in your respiratory system but also your digestive system.

As treatment strategies are becoming more effective, it is becoming more common to pursue pregnancy with an existing diagnosis of cystic fibrosis (CF). Additionally, acupuncture works on a different type of channel and can be effective for obstructive respiratory diseases. And even though it's hereditary, studies have shown that if you have CF, it can still be a viable choice to have a baby. The majority of these pregnancies produce healthy, noncystic fibrosis babies. The severity of your condition is a significant predictor to how well you and baby will fare.

Syncope, Dizziness, and Fainting

Your world may be spinning with the prospect of having a baby, and there might be actual dizziness to physically prove it. Fainting for a moment—called "syncope"—is on the spectrum of dizziness and isn't for the faint of heart (pun intended). Everything is changing, including your circulation. Your blood vessels are more dilated, so although blood flow is increased to baby, it flows a bit slower for you; therefore, your heart beats a little slower, too, which lowers your blood pressure a bit and reduces blood flow to your brain. All of this can cause incidences of dizziness and even fainting. These are pretty common symptoms in the first trimester and even throughout pregnancy.

In the second and third trimesters, your growing uterus puts pressure on and can constrict your blood flow, which is related to why you don't want to lie on your back as your pregnancy progresses—the weight of the baby compresses your *vena cava*, the vein that transports blood from your lower body to your heart (or, when you're lying down, doesn't so much).

The main reasons for dizziness and fainting are structural pressure, low blood sugar, and dehydration. To stave off the smelling salts, wear loose-fitting clothing, position yourself well when you sit or lie down, get up very slowly, snack often (especially on iron-rich foods) and stay hydrated (electrolyte-laced water is the best: see recipe page 37).

If your heart is beating noticeably faster, this may be due to increased fluid volume, which makes the heart work harder, and shortness of breath can be an inevitable and a very normal course throughout pregnancy. However, if it is a regular occurrence accompanied by dizziness or actual passing out, or if you've passed out for more than fifteen minutes at a time, it's important to check in with your care provider and potentially consult with a neurologist and/or cardiologist.

Other symptoms to watch for include chest pain, incontinence, blurry vision, and vaginal bleeding. Any of the above can be normal but can also indicate something that is worth monitoring closely and looking into more comprehensively if it persists or progresses.

Incontinence

Pelvic floor muscle training is often recommended during pregnancy and after birth for the prevention and treatment of incontinence (both urinary and fecal—and yes, this is unfortunately something you may have to look forward to if you're among the one-third of women who experience these symptoms post-birth). You can consider going to Pilates or yoga to address "the core," or start doing traditional Kegel exercises while you are still pregnant.

Kegels involve contracting the pelvic muscles gradually up and back down again, like rungs of a ladder, as if you're squeezing and holding urine in (but don't actually do that, since it can weaken the bladder). Hold each contraction for one breath and gradually increase the rungs. Try to practice ten rounds a day. Since practicing is imperceptible to the casual bystander, you can spice up your day by doing several sets of Kegels while you're doing something banal.

Carpal Tunnel Syndrome

There are a lot of reasons to avoid lifting heavy objects while pregnant, and carpal tunnel is one of them. This pain-in-the-wrist syndrome, often prevalent during pregnancy, can seriously interfere with routine activities. The first indicators can include symptoms such as hand pain or numbness, tingling sensations in your fingers, shooting pain in your forearms, and loss of grip strength or dexterity.

Why is this happening now? Carpal tunnel occurs during pregnancy because with all of the increased pressure and buildup of fluid in your body, there is increased pressure on the nerves that run through your wrists. They are impaired to some extent in virtually all pregnant women during their third trimester. Upper back and neck tension are also implicated, because the seized muscles pinch nerves and further decrease blood circulation to your arms.

Unfortunately, carpal tunnel can persist for months or years after birth, but it usually abates much sooner than that. To help manage your current symptoms and to prepare you for a quick recovery, strategies that I've found helpful are massage; acupuncture; yoga that focuses on the upper back, arms, and wrists; and the occasional need for a wrist splint to provide a little extra stability. Since the symptoms are often worse at night, if carpal tunnel is interfering with your sleep, check out the insomnia section for some extra tips.

Although its effectiveness is debatable, vitamin B6 is often used as a therapy in treatment of carpal tunnel syndrome. This might be because vitamin B6 helps the peripheral nerves and circulatory system, or because it can act as an analgesic (pain reliever) by raising pain thresholds. Regardless, if it works, it works. The typical therapeutic dose for addressing carpal tunnel with B6 is 100 mg a day. During pregnancy, B6 should only be taken for seven days in a row, while monitoring for any side effects such as light sensitivity or skin irritation. If these occur, stop taking B6 immediately; the symptoms should go away immediately. Nausea and heartburn can be symptoms of too much B6 as well, but those might be hard to tease out during pregnancy. Ironically, a very high daily dose of B6 (500 mg a day) can cause nerve damage. So, as I always recommend, before you turn to supplements, start with foods that are rich in B6 such as chicken, hazelnuts, salmon, spinach, sunflower seeds, and yams—and, if needed, then try a supplemental B6, taken alongside a B complex or your prenatal vitamin.

The bright side to carpal tunnel? This is a good time to really indulge in minimizing strenuous tasks and engage people to wait on you. May I suggest a bell?

Vivid Dreams

The record of dreaming and dream interpretation dates back to 4,000 BCE, when dreams were documented on clay tablets, and dreams have been used ever since—including in ancient Greece, Egypt, and China—to elucidate parts of the dreamer's life he or she may not be conscious of. There are some modern studies in neurology, which demonstrate that recalling your dreams relies upon the same mechanisms in the brain as recalling actual memories.

Regardless of this blurred line between waking or sleeping, you're bound to be bleary with wild and vivid dreams during pregnancy, and whether you think of dreaming as a way to learn more about yourself or just as a time to check out for a while, you may want to keep a journal by your bed to record your dreams. It can provide an interesting additional storyline to your pregnancy.

Practical Baby Preparation

Personally, my approach to baby paraphernalia is minimalist, so I've only included the bare essentials on this list. You can, of course, fluff it up with as many things as you need to help you feel comfortable, excited, and prepared. Just bear in mind, there's a tendency to think you need everything right away, but the truth is that for many weeks, all that baby needs is *you* (and some essentials). Once the baby is born, you'll figure the rest out as you go along, so no need to stress yourself out ahead of time.

Bare Essentials Priority Checklist

- Somewhere for baby to sleep (If you are planning to cosleep with your baby, look into cosleeping options for baby's safety.)
- 1-2 blankets for wrapping or swaddling
- Onesies (You'll probably change them multiple times a day, so having a week's worth will minimize constant laundry.)
- Lots of burp cloths (You can use cloth diapers for extra absorbency.)
- Three large boxes of newborn diapers or the equivalent of cloth
- Two diaper covers if using cloth diapers
- Diaper cream
- Unscented baby wipes
- Changing pad
- Socks or booties, pajamas, hat
- Infant car seat, installed
- Baby thermometer
- If you're breastfeeding: pump, milk storage bags
- If you're not breastfeeding: eight containers of formula (see resource section for a good quality formula suggestion) and glass or BPA-free 4-ounce plastic bottles with slow flow nipples
- Unscented, perfume/dye-free laundry detergent
- Humidifier (optional but recommended—especially if you live in a dry climate or your baby will be born during the winter)

Birth Plan

While it's a good idea not to overly anticipate exactly how your birth will go, a birth plan is a wonderful way to dream about your labor and the birth of your child and can be an important medium for clarifying an idea of how you'd like to approach the birth decisions you may be faced with. As you're

The Birth Plan

My approach to a birth plan isn't the standard list of questions about step-by-step planning. In some ways I think that method can set you up for feelings of disappointment or confusion, because the truth is, birth goes how it goes. It doesn't mean you shouldn't be educated and map out what you'd like or not like—such as epidural or no epidural, photos or no photos of the actual birth—or abandon hope that your birth will go exactly the way you want. It's possible that it will, but it's also important to cultivate a lot of room for encountering the unknown and not only coping, but emerging confident that you had the best process you could have.

Take some time to mull over the following questions. You may be surprised at what you come up with.

1. When you imagine meeting your baby, what does that feel like? How does he or she feel in your arms? What does it feel like to gaze into each other's eyes? What other images or emotions come up in this fantasy?

2. Do you imagine saying anything in particular?

3. What does the thought of being out of control bring up for you?

4. Can you imagine being wild? What does that look like for you?

5. Do have any fears or feelings of embarrassment when you imagine the birth scenario? Can you imagine letting those go? What would you need to help you let go?

6. Where in your body can you imagine letting go of more tension (even if it seems unrelated to birth)?

7. What fears or anxieties do you have about birth? Can you find where those feelings reside in your body? What do they need to be soothed?

8. What is one thing you absolutely don't want to happen during birth? If this very thing happened, what would you do to cope?

9. Who would you like at your birth? Be honest with yourself.

10. Who are you going to have with you to represent your desires for your birth and interpret the choices for you as you go along in the birth process?

11. Do you trust and have confidence in your midwife or obstetrician? Is there anything you need to ask them or of them before birth?

Can you tuck your answers to all of these questions and the feelings you've connected with away somewhere in your body to draw on if you need some inspiration during the birth process? Can you tell a person who is supporting you during birth to remind you of this "plan" during the birth?

Since birth just goes how it goes, I would suggest that you intend these questions to provoke a deep sense of inner guidance in you and stimulate your preferences while leaving plenty of room for possibility.

sketching out your desires, remember to stay with the idea of flexibility around all the many unknowns that may arise during birth. Be able to trust and invest in the team around you to safely support your preferences.

Birthing Choices

There is a lot of discussion about natural birth choices versus routine medical interventions for birth, including controversies around the rationale for an increasing rate of caesarean sections in some hospitals. Labor and delivery can be a beautiful experience. Although nobody knows exactly how their birth will go, it can be an empowering experience to think about the elements of your birth process that are important to you and become educated about appropriate ways to modify your original intentions, should medical necessity warrant it. Knowing the difference between medical necessity and convenience is key. Having a competent doula at a hospital birth can free you up to safely explore your birth preferences.

Hospital births are the obvious choice for many, and each hospital has its own aspects and offerings for you to explore. Here are some other birth choices, as well as elements to consider utilizing to enhance your birth process—whether at the hospital or at home. Remember, there is no right or wrong. No matter what or how you choose to approach birth, the important thing is that you feel nurtured and safe.

Nurse Midwife in a Hospital Setting

Certified nurse midwives (CNMs) are trained in both nursing and midwifery and are certified by the American College of Nurse-Midwives (ACNM). CNMs function as primary care providers in hospital settings or birthing centers for women who are not in a high-risk birth category. Nurse midwives work in close collaboration with the OBGYNs at their facility. So, you get the full-fledged Western environment with a slant toward holistic birth methods.

Birthing Center

The ABC's of alternative birthing centers are that they offer family-centered, home-like, low-technology maternity care. They are free-standing centers—not associated with hospitals—and like any practice based on midwifery, screen to rule out accepting women who are anticipated to have complicated pregnancies or deliveries that require more sophisticated, hospital-based technology (such as twins or breech presentation). If you're considering giving birth at a birth center, this is something to keep in mind.

Home Birth

For many centuries, of course, births always took place at home. Hospitals with modern technology have enabled safer births for many women and newborns who may have otherwise had less favorable outcomes, but in the last twenty years, many women have begun to revisit their interest in home-birth. They choose home births for reasons such as privacy, comfort, convenience, cultural continuity, and finances, and to ultimately to have a hand in orchestrating their birth and birth attendants in the way they see fit.

Midwives who attend home births are either certified midwives or direct-entry midwives, and they have a larger scope of education and tools under their belt than most people realize. Plus, they typically collaborate with a back-up physician to account for any potential emergencies that may require transport to a hospital during birth. For some, this model can be the best of both worlds.

If you are not in the category of a high-risk birth, the medical literature continues to acknowledge that home births attended by a well-trained midwife typically require less medical intervention and are not associated with higher risks than hospital births. Although there is extensive documentation to support the safety of choosing home birth, each pregnancy and birth carries its own unique parameters and potential risks. Home birth is an extensive topic that deserves to be well researched by you and discussed with health care providers that you trust to best determine if it is the right choice for you.

See the resources section under midwives to links for further exploration of safety and resources for home birth options.

Methods and Tools to Enhance Hospital or Home Births

Water Birth

The American Pregnancy Association recognizes that there are many benefits to water births. Whether you actually deliver in the birthing tub or not, it can be a great tool to ease your labor—literal levity. Since the baby has been floating around in amniotic fluid, a warm tub of water can be a natural and gentle transition. The buoyancy can help your own transitions with positioning and labor stages as well. Bathing is an age-old way to reduce stress, and performing this ablution during birth can soothe and wash away some of your tensions and contribute ease to your birth.

As with anything, there are some potential risks with water birthing that include the baby gasping and inhaling water (which is rare, since their reflex is only to inhale upon exposure to air) or the umbilical cord tearing while baby is being lifted from the water.

A water birth is not a good choice if any of the following conditions exist:

- Bleeding disorders
- Breech presentation
- Copious amounts of meconium
- Pre-existing herpes (enhances the risk of transmission to baby)
- Preeclampsia
- Toxemia

You can rent birth tubs and have them installed, either at home or at the hospital (if permitted), and some centers already have them available. If you're using a birth tub at a hospital, start the process well in advance of your birth to make sure that you can accommodate all of the red tape.

Overall, there is little difference in danger between babies delivered in water versus out of water. So sink into whatever choice is right for you.

Doula Support

The word *doula* originated from a Greek word meaning "female servant." In a more modern sense, doulas provide a wonderful service to women before and during labor, by offering coaching and guidance on self-care throughout your process. A well-trained and experienced doula can also be a great intermediary between understanding and assessing the need for medical interventions in a hospital setting as well as helping you and your partner effectively collaborate during the birth (read: show partner where to rub, and so on).

A postpartum doula can be a delightful and arguably essential addition for your first few days to weeks after birth. They help with cooking, lactation consulting, and monitoring your postpartum recovery, and they will take the night shift so that you can get some sleep. It can be very reassuring to have a competent resource around in the middle of the night as you're figuring it all out.

Hypnobirthing

Hypnosis has actually been used in obstetrics for over a hundred years, and the modern idea of hypnobirthing continues to be a soothing and efficacious choice for many women approaching and interfacing with their ideas or fears about birth. Hypnobirthing is less about avoiding pain and more about retraining your relationship to pain or sensation. This is a method that aims to connect the mind-body communication so that you really can dream up your birth. This can also be a great resource for women predisposed to anxiety—regardless of the normalcy of having anxiety when initially anticipating birth. This addition to your birth prep can be a great coping strategy and for such a minor intervention, potentially significantly enhance your experience of birth.

A Note on Vaginal Birth After Caesarean Section (VBAC)

Caesarean delivery is the most common operating-room procedure in the United States. But just because you needed or opted for a C-section in a prior birth doesn't necessarily mean that you need or want a C-section this time. If you've previously had a Caesarean section and you want to aim for a vaginal delivery with this pregnancy, it's called a Vaginal Birth After Caesarean, or VBAC.

Vaginal birth is, of course, more likely to injure your sphincter or cause trauma to your perineum than a C-section, but the benefits of VBACs include:

- Less scarring to the uterus (in case you may want to have more children)

- Reduced risk of infection

- Quicker recovery time after delivery, which can enhance the way you are able to care for your newborn and will reduce your hospital time

- Potential physiological benefits to the baby, including some immune transmission which occurs when passing through the birth canal, which may contribute to a full spectrum of hormone release and make breastfeeding a bit easier (although, many women can successfully breastfeed after C-sections as well)

- If you and your doctor are in agreement about the possibility of a VBAC, you'll enter a "trial of labor"—meaning you'll start out with the goal of averting the need for another C-section and see how it goes.

Delivery Prep Strategies

Anticipation of your birth is heightening, and you may be curious about how to prepare. There are many strategies, but the most important is always to take great care of yourself through nutrition, exercise, and rest and to find the balance between preparing for a set of unknowns and surrendering to an inevitable process that will simply go how it will go. Know that the healthier you are, the better it will most likely go.

How you approach childbirth is a choice. How it actually happens may be a bit out of your hands. Whatever you're feeling, focus on working with your feelings, understanding the origin of any fears you may have, and examining your level of readiness. Keep staying with yourself—nobody else's idea of how this will be for you is relevant. Each birth is incredibly different, and many women experience relatively pleasurable births. And know that nature has a wonderful built-in mechanism for helping you forget any trauma as soon as you see your new baby. This will imbue you with stamina and joy to focus on the new life you brought into this world.

Parenting Tips

At this point in your pregnancy, you may be thinking beyond the actual birth to the time when you will be a parent. There is no tried-and-true manual for parenting, but there is emerging evidence to support certain healthy parenting techniques. The best advice I've ever heard, which seems to be full of good foundational suggestions, comes from the research of John Gottman, a professor emeritus of psychology at the University of Washington. His books *Raising An Emotionally Intelligent Child: The Heart of Parenting* and *And Baby Makes Three: The Six-Step Plan for Preserving Marital Intimacy and Rekindling Romance After Baby Arrives* delve into keeping the parental unit strong and healthy to successfully transfer emotional stability to your child and ultimately have a well-balanced family unit.

Checklist for Month Seven

- Investigate birth strategies and choices.
- Develop your "birth plan."
- Enlist a doula if you're going that route.

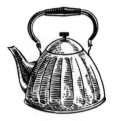

Month Eight
Preparing

WEEK THIRTY-THREE

· Baby has had a big growth spurt from last week to 18 inches and 5 pounds.

· Eyes are opening and closing during sleep and wake cycles.

· Bones are becoming denser.

· Baby is developing more coordinated breathing patterns.

WEEK THIRTY-FOUR

· Baby weighs in about the same a last week.

· He or she is urinating about a pint a day.

· Fingernails and toenails have grown in.

WEEK THIRTY-FIVE

· Baby is still about 18 inches and 5 pounds.

· Hearing is fully developed.

· Liver is now processing waste.

· If you're having a boy, his testes are descending.

....

WEEK THIRTY-SIX

· Baby is holding at 18 inches and 5 pounds.

· Skin is smoothing out.

· Gums are more rigid.

· Baby's immune system has absorbed your antibodies and is prepared for the world.

....

East-West Fetal Development

This month is associated with the Chinese Large Intestine system. On a functional Western level, the large intestine is about assimilating nutrients and eliminating waste. This month, you and your baby continue to absorb nutrition in preparation for baby to move out. This can be a good time to contemplate what you need to hold onto and what you can let go of in order to assist you in surrendering to the birth process with as few impediments as possible. It's also worth noting that having a bowel movement is a normal part of the active birth process. So, if you knew this and had any particular reservations, work on letting them go, and if you didn't know this, now you do!

Bed Rest

Bed rest, of course, doesn't just mean *spa day*. It is a medical recommendation that means really only get up to pee and is typically instituted in order to prevent preterm delivery. So, the news isn't usually celebrated, but if you've been put on bed rest, take full advantage of this time (however long it may seem) to catch up on quiet and productive activities that you may not have the luxury of doing amidst the normal bustle—and certainly not once baby arrives. Comfort yourself with the knowledge that you are in the first throes of parenthood, putting aspects of your agenda aside to accommodate someone else's well-being.

Inflammatory Bowel Syndrome, Crohn's Disease, and Ulcerative Colitis

Inflammatory bowel syndrome (IBS), Crohn's disease (CD), and ulcerative colitis (UC) are all gastrointestinal (GI) conditions that can include, with some variances, bowel discomfort and changes, abdominal pain, and abdominal bloating.

Brain-gut interactions are increasingly recognized as paired mechanisms in GI issues, so mind-body medicine such as hypnotherapy and meditation can be useful approaches. Acupuncture has also been studied in the treatment of gastrointestinal symptoms. It works on the brain-gut disturbances and influences the bowels and gut in terms of cramping and acid secretion.

These conditions can be very stressful for you, and they can be stressful for baby too. Some studies have shown that nutritional approaches such as the use of probiotics are not only a possible preventative agent against your GI dysfunctions, but can also provide aid for your baby's potential stressors. Probiotics have specifically been shown to modulate the sensitive gut characteristics of IBS.

Probiotic-rich foods include kefir, miso, sauerkraut, and yogurt with live cultures. Incorporating soluble fiber in the form of whole grains, fruits, and vegetables can instigate some relief as well. Also, consider approaching your diet with overall anti-inflammatory strategies (see the Easy Anti-Inflammatory Eating Plan for Candida sidebar on pages 110–111) and identifying foods that may exacerbate your condition, such a wheat or dairy. In other words, *listen to your gut.*

Headaches

Most headaches during pregnancy are just headaches. The management is usually the same as when you're not pregnant: eat, drink (water, not martinis), and sleep. However, those predisposed to migraines are very sensitive to the hormonal milieu of pregnancy, and if you had migraines before pregnancy, they might very well appear during pregnancy with different patterns than you're used to. Migraines without auras usually benefit from the spike in estrogen and the decrease in normal monthly hormonal fluctuations. But migraines *with* auras often don't improve during pregnancy.

There are also some links between migraines and the potential for an increased risk of developing gestational hypertension or preeclampsia. If your migraines are on the rise during pregnancy, be aggressive about managing your well-being through nutrition and exercise and keep an eye on your blood pressure. Acupuncture works wonders for most migraines.

The silver lining: after delivery, breastfeeding has a bit of a protective effect against migraines.

Baby's Position

Baby's position prior to birth is called *the presentation of the fetus*. As the baby is getting ready for her big debut, she may move around right up until the very last moment, but when the moment does come, some positions are more ideal than others.

The most common and ideal position for labor is called *cephalic presentation*. This is when the baby is head-down, facing your back, with her chin tucked into her chest. If your baby is already settled in this position at this point, she'll likely remain here.

Some other positions may indicate a more complicated birth and sometimes call for a cesarean delivery—although remember, babies do still move and adjust during the birth process.

- *Occiput or cephalic posterior*, or "sunny side up," is when the baby is head down but facing your abdomen.

- In a *breech presentation*, the baby's bottom is down. Coming through the birth canal in this way could increase the chance of forming an umbilical cord loop that could cause injury to the baby during a vaginal birth, but there are still opportunities for baby to turn right up until the end of your pregnancy (although, as space gets tighter, it does decrease the likelihood).

- In a *footling breech*, one or both of the baby's feet are at the lowest portion of your uterus. This is a complicated presentation because of the potential impact on the umbilical cord.

- A *transverse lie* is when the baby is lengthwise in the uterus, making it likely that the shoulder will enter the pelvis first. Most babies in this position need some good maneuvering during the birth process or to be delivered via C-section.

For repositioning, there's all sorts of folksy advice out there—somersaults in pools, playing music for your uterus, shining a flashlight up there, etc. Honestly, I always encourage you to do whatever does no harm and feels right for you, but the methods that tend to work the most reliably are:

- Your midwife or physician manually tries to shift the baby. This process should be carefully monitored in case it causes complications.

- A Chinese medicine technique of applying an herbal application called *moxibustion* on a particular point on the little toe has a lot of backing for helping to turn a breech presentation. Start this with your acupuncturist as early in your third trimester as possible.

It is also very important to remember that often, when baby doesn't turn or shift despite all of your good intentions and coaxing for a vaginal birth, it may be and often is for a good reason. For instance, the umbilical cord may be wrapped around baby in a way that would make shifting dangerous. The most common instance of this is a nuchal loop—the cord wrapped around the baby's neck. There's really nothing you can do about a cord knot other than monitor the normal activity of your baby. So, trust in your wisdom, but also the baby's.

Real, Uncomfortable Weight Gain and Fatigue

It's important to revisit the concept of fatigue throughout pregnancy. It was probably your central focus during the first trimester, but it can be a growing frustration again at this stage. Some women do still walk marathons in their seventh month, but most are just trying to get through their day awake.

It's normal to be tired. You are lugging around a lot of extra weight and still, as always during pregnancy, actively contributing to your baby's growth. There's no way around this feeling, and giving yourself permission to rest as much as possible is great preparation for the upcoming work of labor, delivery, and breastfeeding. If you feel like your weight is out of bounds, refer back to the section on healthy weight gain to help you further assess other strategies.

Back, Sciatic, and Leg Pain

Because enough wasn't going on already, let's add back and ligament pain into the mix! Fifty percent of pregnant women experience some kind of back pain. In fact, it's the most common reason that pregnancy interferes with work, especially if you have a job that requires either sustained sitting or standing—in other words, pretty much every job. In combination with the structural aspects of carrying more weight and all the physical compensations that start to happen in order to balance this new load, there are hormones (of course) at play that can predispose you to being more susceptible to a lack of stability in your ligaments, and therefore joints—especially pelvic joints.

The Role of Relaxin and Its Effect on the Pelvis and Pelvic Girdle Pain

Relaxin is secreted by the corpus luteum and the placenta and is one of the prevalent hormones during pregnancy. *Relaxin* is a bit of a euphemistic name, because it's less like something that helps you kick your feet up and relax and more like something that turns your connective tissue into noodles and creates general instability in your musculoskeletal system—although that's certainly a good reason to put your feet up too.

Relaxin specifically targets the pubic symphysis and sacroiliac joints. It is helpful later on to assist with cervical ripening and relaxing and opening your pelvis to prepare for birth, but in the meantime, it can predispose you to low back and pelvic aches and pains.

Then there's pelvic girdle pain, which presents as a persistent pain in the front and/or back of your pelvis. This pain can radiate across your hip joints and thighbones. Symptoms can start as early as the first trimester, at labor, or even begin *after* birth.

The Tug on the Round Ligaments

The round ligaments, which connect the uterus to the abdomen, bear more weight as your baby grows, and this strain can cause a tugging sensation—like a rope anchoring a sailboat on a windy day—that can feel like pulling, spasms, or cramps. This type of pain is usually found more on your right side because of the general uterine growth pattern.

The Shooting Pain of Sciatica

Sciatica is quite common during pregnancy. Sciatic pain is typically characterized by a one-sided (although, it can be both) shooting, burning pain or tingling sensation from your low back through your gluteus muscles and down your leg, and sometimes all the way into your toes.

Sciatica usually flares up in the third trimester, when baby is positioning himself for birth, which means your little bundle is resting on your nerve bundles. At term, the uterus weighs approximately two and a half pounds, and the baby adds about six and a half more pounds. (If it makes you feel any better, the largest baby recorded in medical literature was twenty-five pounds!) This weight puts direct pressure on the nerve roots in your back—hence, back pain. Unfortunately, severe vomiting earlier in pregnancy can sometimes trigger sciatic pain too.

Pelvic Discomfort and Symphysis Pubis Dysfunction (SPD)

Baby is preparing for her descent down the birth canal by settling lower and lower into your uterus. You may have heard the term "the baby has dropped." This refers to baby's head engaging your cervix and comes with some pretty sizeable pelvic, hip, back, and all-over discomfort. It also comes with the exciting news that you're almost ready to meet your baby!

Even if you're not having trouble with any of the above, there's also the mechanics of your abdominal muscles that must stretch to accommodate growth, which causes muscle fatigue and an extra load on your spine.

The most important factor that aggravates low-back and pelvic pain during pregnancy is simply the progression of a normal, growing pregnancy. Many aches and pains may be inevitable throughout certain stages of your pregnancy, but some effective strategies to manage them and possibly reduce the aggravation include pelvic-tilt exercises (which can reduce ligament pain intensity and pain duration) and acupuncture. In the case of the latter, there's lots of research to show its efficacy in relieving low-back and pelvic pain during pregnancy without adverse side effects, plus it can increase your capacity for some physical activity and help diminish the need for other interventions, which is a big advantage during pregnancy.

For some manual release, prenatal massage with an experienced practitioner can be incredibly beneficial. Other suggestions for relief and strengthening your postural support are a warm hot water bottle on your pubic bone (unless you notice that this creates more feelings of inflammation—then ice it instead), regular stretching and exercise (to whatever extent is available), prenatal Pilates, regular physical therapy, and swimming. A pelvic belt can also apply some compression, which makes you feel less loosey-goosey, and even though it seems like a chastity belt, clearly it's not.

Often, enduring pain for a sustained amount of time becomes not about the pain itself, but more about the ways that pain interferes with daily functioning, sleep, and mental well-being. If you're experiencing pain in your pregnancy, this is an opportune time for some nonrigorous breathing and relaxation exercises. Try to avoid prolonged walking or standing—there's nothing like a midday rest to help you regenerate. The Kidneys control the bones in Chinese medicine and rest fuels the Kidney system and helps you not be literally bone tired.

Differentiating Between Braxton-Hicks and Labor Contractions

Most people are curious what Braxton-Hicks contractions are. First, let's talk about who Braxton Hicks *was*. John Braxton Hicks was an obstetrician in the mid-1800s who was also a pioneer in midwifery. He was the first one to describe the rhythmic contractions of the uterus that occur throughout pregnancy (now simply known as Braxton-Hicks).

Most of my patients ask me how they'll be able to tell the difference between a "real" contraction and Braxton-Hicks contractions. The simple advice is that *you'll just know*. Until you have a labor-related contraction, you might think Braxton-Hicks are "real" contractions, but when you have an actual contraction, you'll quickly feel the difference.

Braxton-Hicks, or preparatory contractions, *are* true contractions in the sense that oxytocin is stimulating the uterus to contract, just like it does during labor, but these contractions are not strong enough to elicit actual labor. Braxton-Hicks are simply a normal part of the body's readying for labor. They don't occur at regular intervals and often dissipate with positional or activity changes. I think of them as an erratic exercise routine—your body is alternately practicing for labor and then getting distracted and going about its day—then realizing again that it's in training, and doing a little "sprint."

Remember, your uterus is used to expelling things during menstruation. Now, it is also preparing itself to assist with birth. Incidentally, Dr. Hicks also had a large collection of Wedgwood china, so sit back and relax with some tea while you commemorate how this normal symptom will eventually contribute to shaping your birth process.

Some signs of actual labor onset (more on this in month nine) include contractions that feel like vaginal or menstrual cramps every five to ten minutes or less (more than five contractions in an hour), consistent pain and/or pressure in your back or lower abdomen or pelvis, leaking fluid, and nausea, vomiting, or diarrhea.

It can be confusing, and it's okay to not be sure. If you need some help clarifying what's going on, call your provider. Your safety and preparation for birth are always the most important thing.

Preterm Labor

Ready or not, baby may be coming. Labor anytime before your thirty-seventh week is considered preterm labor. It includes symptoms of—you guessed it—labor! These may be all or some of the symptoms you experience:

- Contractions at least every ten minutes
- Persistent backache
- Feeling of baby pushing down on pelvis (because he is)
- Discharge or profuse amounts of water leaking from your vagina (possibly premature rupture of the membranes)
- Spotting or bleeding
- Vomiting and/or diarrhea

Obviously, you and your delivery team will do everything you can to keep the baby in for as long as possible, but if you're after thirty-four weeks, the evidence points to delivery usually being the most successful route in the face of other threats. Additionally, once your water breaks, you are far more susceptible to infections such as chorioamnionitis—an inflammation of the fetal membranes from a bacterial infection, which is mostly from bacteria coming from the vagina into the uterus. In general, this is why not too many vaginal exams are done later in pregnancy or during labor when the cervix is more open.

During pregnancy, there is a reduction in your stores of an omega-3 fatty acid called Docosahexaenoic acid (DHA), and the synthesis of long chain polyunsaturated fatty acids (LCPUFA) in the baby and placenta is low. So supplementing with up to 1 gram per day of omega-3 LCPUFAs (I recommend erring toward walnuts or flaxseed oil versus sardines since methylmercury exposure from fish can do more harm than good during pregnancy) has shown to potentially increase birth weight. So if you do need to deliver early, baby is at least fattening up! Another nice by-product of this type of supplementation is that it also tends to reduce allergies in babies (and susceptible immunity can of course be an issue with preterm babies).

See No Cons to Probiotics on page 77 to read a bit about their potential effect for preventing preterm labor as well.

The Art of Flattering Photos

If you read this as "fattening photos," I get it. You may not be feeling your most svelte or photogenic, but try to remember that what's making you feel somewhat enormous is that healthy baby inside of you. Photography during this time is not to memorialize your idea of your body you once knew, but to capture a time when your body was doing exactly what it was designed to do—and doing it beautifully. There are many wonderful ways to accentuate the beauty of this time. So, be creative with commemorating your body and this important stage in your life.

Checklist for Month Eight

- Stock up on household and baby supplies (see Bare Essentials Priority Checklist on page 155) such as toiletries and natural, unscented laundry detergent.
- Tie up loose ends.
- Make arrangements for your absence at work.
- Organize financial obligations.

- Finalize your intentions/plan for birth.
- Arrange help for after birth.
- Install baby's car seat.
- Make sure all your ducks are in a row since you're now in the zone of "anything goes."

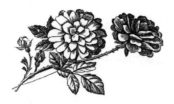

Month Nine
Releasing

WEEK THIRTY-SEVEN

- Baby is 19.5 inches and 7.5 pounds.
- You are officially full term!

WEEK THIRTY-EIGHT

- Baby is 19.5 inches and 7.5 ounces.
- Baby's head is now filling out your abdomen.
- Head hair is visible on ultrasound (if they're growing it—plenty of babies are cute and bald).
- Baby is shedding the vernix caseosa.
- Lungs are continuing to mature and produce surfactant.

WEEK THIRTY-NINE

- Baby is 19.5 inches and 7.5 ounces.
- Fingernails and toenails are completely grown.
- New skin cells are beginning to generate.
- Brain is still rapidly developing.
- More fat has been deposited to ready baby for insulation in the world.

....

WEEK FORTY

· Baby is 19.5 inches and 7.5 ounces.

· All of baby's bones have solidified (except for the skull, which remains relatively soft in order to make the journey through the birth canal).

· Baby is engaged in birth position and may be on the way out!

....

East-West Fetal Development

Month nine is associated with the Chinese Kidney system, which is analogous to the endocrine system. This month is a culmination of all of the reproductive processes that have transpired from conception until now, and the Kidneys as much as they are responsible for holding the baby in, also govern the letting go. The element associated with the Kidneys is water. This is a time of going with the flow, so to speak. Very literally, your water will break this month to pave the way for the passage of your baby.

The Kidneys are the most fundamental system in Chinese medicine. This system gives rise to immunity and genetics—all things that you have passed onto your baby. The Kidneys are also associated with winter, so no matter what season it is, this is a good time to go inward and be as dormant as possible in order to build your reserves for birth and beyond.

Hair and Nails

Most people think that hair thickens during pregnancy, but what actually happens is perhaps a little less glamorous: hair just falls out much slower because the increased estrogen delays hair loss. That's why there's a mass exodus of your hair during your postpartum period—you're not actually going bald, just resuming normal hair loss and making up for the ones that were spared during pregnancy.

In Chinese medicine, head hair is associated with the Kidney as well. While you're storing up all of your reserves during birth, the head hair reflects this with its thickness and shine. After birth, the Kidney system is drained a bit, so the hair falls out. It's important to nourish and support this Kidney system throughout pregnancy with rest and good food in order

....

HAIR AND NAIL RESTORATION TEA

4 cups filtered water

3 tablespoons each dried oat straw, bamboo leaf, and horsetail*

Directions

Combine herbs and water in a glass jar and let soak at room temperature overnight. Strain liquid and keep in fridge. Drink one cup a day.

NOTE: Do not use horsetail herb if you take an ACE inhibitor for high blood pressure or if you have congestive heart failure, as this combination can cause an excessive accumulation of potassium.

* See the resource section for ingredients for this tea.

....

to set you up for a healthy postpartum recovery and equip you with all the resources you'll need for yourself and baby.

Nails do actually grow faster during pregnancy, but can also become more brittle or develop grooves. This echoes back to our discussion about the Chinese idea of blood deficiency in pregnancy. So this can be a great indicator to boost up on iron-rich, or blood-building foods.

Inflammatory Rheumatic Diseases

Rheumatoid arthritis, ankylosing spondylitis. and systemic lupus erythematosus are all conditions characterized by chronic inflammation, joint pain, and swelling. The body's immune system can also become hyperactive in these conditions, leading to further attack on healthy tissue.

Pregnant women with any of these conditions are capable of having uncomplicated pregnancies, but since the risk for complications is increased, it is advisable to enlist the cooperation of a rheumatologist and nephrologist in addition to your gynecologist. An acupuncturist is a great addition to this team as well.

For all of the above conditions, anti-inflammatory eating strategies can help with management. Combining the following foods in your dishes can sprinkle some potent anti-inflammatory and immune-boosting action into your meals:

- Basil
- Blueberries
- Celery
- Cinnamon
- Ginger root
- Oregano
- Parsley
- Rosemary
- Shitake mushrooms

Scoliosis

Outside of its potential to increase discomfort as you start to carry more weight, scoliosis has little correlation to difficult pregnancies—or even an increased need for caesarean delivery. But to bolster and strengthen your bones, I suggest you eat mineral-rich broths and calcium-rich foods throughout your pregnancy and find a balance between maintaining mobility and good rest.

Multiple Sclerosis

Multiple sclerosis (MS) is the most commonly acquired neurological disorder affecting young women, but the good news is that it does not usually have a negative impact on pregnancy. Some studies suggest that estrogen exposure during pregnancy may even have protective effects against the disease's progression.

Other studies indicate that women with MS do have a slightly increased risk for having small-for-gestational-age newborns, but most babies of MS women do not develop MS themselves.

However, if you are on immunomodulatory therapy for MS, you should discontinue it before conception or as soon as you find out (though low doses of prednisone may still be okay).

Coming to Terms with Your Readiness

In 2014, the American College of Obstetricians and Gynecologists (ACOG) released a statement refining some of its previous definitions around full-term birth and estimated dates of delivery (EDD). An excerpt from the ACOG statement reads "Babies born between thirty-nine and forty weeks, six days have the best health outcomes, compared with babies born before or after this period. This distinct time period is now referred to as 'full term.'"

Of course, the above parameters don't account for your own feelings of readiness, but anchoring yourself in the thought of what's optimal for your baby's health will continue to give you stamina to endure these last weeks. You're almost there! Most babies come when they're ready—and most are ready within the timeframe above.

While you are patiently or otherwise waiting for the moment to arrive, see if there are any remaining ways you can nurture yourself and indulge in a little more "me" time. If you're able to maintain some regular, gentle exercise, all the better for continuing your preparation. Swimming, in particular, can be fantastic right now. Most importantly, rest up. You'll need all of your stamina for birth and beyond, and you'll reminisce soon about the opportunity to nap at will.

As uncomfortable as you may be, try to find ways to enjoy and revel in these last moments of your pregnancy, and know that babies typically come when they're good and ready.

Nesting

Before the baby arrives is the best time to get your home to a place that makes you feel comfortable and cozy. After birth, you'll be grateful to have your home ready to receive not just baby, but you.

I recommend lining up some help with food and daily duties, or even creating your own food stores of the stuff you love to eat that's geared toward nourishing you in your postpartum phase. Refer to month ten for some recipes that you can prepare in advance and freeze.

Evaluating Birth Interventions

When evaluating birth interventions such as epidurals and C-sections, the first factor in your decision is of course your own and your baby's safety. I'll present some information about potential risks, but remember that there are also numerous advantages to any of these interventions, depending on your unique situation and needs. Always weigh the information below against your own value system and your evaluation with your healthcare providers.

Primary obstetrical interventions during labor and birth include electronic fetal monitoring (EFM), epidural analgesia, labor induction, two types of delivery instruments (forceps and vacuum), and caesarean section (See more on C-section and VBAC on page 161).

Electronic Fetal Monitoring

Electronic Fetal Monitoring (EFM) is done with elastic belts that use Doppler technology to tell you more about what's happening with your baby during labor, specifically with changes in the heartbeat. The disadvantage is that it can restrict your movement and ability for positional changes during labor, which can potentially interfere with the progress of labor. This process can also be done through periodic auscultation, or listening.

Epidural

About 50 percent of women who give birth at hospitals choose epidurals for pain relief. An epidural is a local anesthetic that significantly dampens, but doesn't usually completely diminish, sensations by blocking nerve impulses that govern the lower half of your body. In order to decrease the medication dose that's required for the local injection, epidurals are often combined with narcotics or other medications to prolong the epidural's effect.

You can also get a "walking epidural," which is an initial injection of pain relievers and a catheter that will enable easy placement of an epidural later, if it becomes necessary.

Epidurals can cause your blood pressure to drop and confine you to one position, which may ultimately slow or stall labor and potentially lead to interventions such as a C-section, but on the other hand, they can also allow you to rest and cope. Many women have positive experiences with epidurals, reporting that it allows them to enjoy the birth of their baby. As with any of these aspects of pregnancy and birth, whether or not to get an epidural is a very personal decision made on the backdrop of your life, your unique definitions of well-being and the actual course of your birth.

Forceps and Vacuum

In experienced hands, forceps or the vacuum method can be tools to help reposition the baby for a vaginal delivery and potentially avert the need for C-section. These two interventions are comparable to each other in terms of safety, and the overall safety for successful birth is very good—the controversy being potential damage to the baby in the process.

Labor Induction

Labor induction to promote uterine contractions is common in 30 percent of pregnancies. You and your healthcare provider should make the assessment together about whether to continue to wait for natural labor or utilize an induction method, but some evaluations that may help your decision-making process include:

- A fetal nonstress test to assess if the baby is receiving enough oxygen
- Stability of your blood pressure
- Sufficient amniotic fluid levels (low amniotic fluid is called oligohydramnios and too much is called polyhydramnios)
- Whether your amniotic fluid membrane, or "water," has broken

Abnormalities in any of these areas can be legitimate reasons to consider natural, manual, or medication-based labor induction methods.

Natural Labor Induction

Some natural induction options which can be effective for safely kick-starting labor are acupuncture, transcutaneous nerve stimulation (TENS), and intercourse with ejaculation of sperm—all of which promote the release of prostaglandins, which are in part responsible for cervical ripening. Additionally, nipple stimulation via massage, sucking, using a breast pump, or a warm compress for an hour three times a day helps stimulate oxytocin (a hormone necessary for uterine contractions).

There are also a few age-old plant-based approaches to helping labor along. The most widely used is evening primrose oil: two 500 mg capsules taken twice a day, plus one capsule inserted as a vaginal suppository at night beginning at week thirty-six may contribute to cervical ripening.

Castor oil has also been used since ancient times to induce labor. It induces prostaglandin stimulation through its laxative and uterine-relaxant effects, but it also contains ricin, which is a potent toxin. I personally don't feel this is worth the benefit of the prostaglandin stimulation that you can get in safer ways through the above modalities.

Black cohosh and blue cohosh are also common remedies, but have been associated with some adverse effects. Black cohosh, although it can relax the uterine muscles, contains salicylic acid (the same compound found in aspirin), so it can contribute to an increased risk of bleeding, both herbs may contribute to elevated liver enzymes (which is something usually monitored during late stages of pregnancy), and interfere with the way the body processes other herbs and supplements you may be taking. If you are working with a midwife, they will be able to advise you about these methods.

Manual Labor Induction

Manual labor interventions, usually done by a midwife or physician, include rupturing the membranes—a manual way to help the water break. The mechanism is similar to some of the natural options in that local pressure stimulates the release of prostaglandins. Most studies show that this is most effective when combined with oxytocin.

The risks associated with rupturing the membranes include infection, abnormal bleeding, and placental disruption.

You can also opt for a hygroscopic dilator—basically a balloon-like device that expands the cervix and provides mechanical pressure. There are natural versions, such as Laminaria japonicum (a seaweed), and synthetic versions, such as Lamicel.

Medication-Based Labor Induction

Pharmacologic agents useful for cervical ripening and labor induction include prostaglandins, misoprostol, mifepristone, relaxin, and oxytocin (also known as Pitocin). These are mostly used when the cervix is already ripe.

In the broad research of low-risk pregnancies, medication-base labor induction shows a higher correlation with the need for the use of either forceps, vacuum, or C-section—and higher rates of episiotomies with more severe tearing. Additionally, mothers who receive labor pain medications (which are often combined with induction drugs) are more likely to report a delayed onset of lactation, regardless of delivery method.

If you choose the medication-based route and have any negative associations or physical repercussions from your birth, know that every mother does the best she can during birth, and that it is impossible to predict the outcome, despite your best decision-making efforts. With the help of the ones you trust, make the best decision that you can make, and strategize about how to move on from there and continue to have the postpartum experience and long life ahead of you and your baby that you desire.

Group B Strep (GBS)

If you've had a history of recurrent yeast infections or urinary tract infections, premature labor, or water breaking before contractions start—or if you have already had a baby who became infected with group B strep (GBS)—you may be particularly predisposed GBS. A simple vaginal culture can be done anywhere from twenty-six to thirty-six weeks to determine if you are positive. I recommend doing it closer to the thirty-six-week mark, since things can change in the last weeks of pregnancy, and that will give you more current information prior to birth.

But group B strep is a tricky one, because it is often a part of normal vaginal flora. You don't necessarily want to jump to advanced interventions such as C-sections just because GBS is present, since only about 1 percent of newborns actually contract it from the active mother.

If you have a propensity toward yeast or urinary tract infections, in addition to good hygiene, the best prevention you can try is to bolster your immune system with probiotics and rest. As long as your water hasn't broken, you can also use a vaginal suppository of goldenseal (one of nature's antibiotics) each evening, beginning at week thirty-four.

If you are positive for group B strep, it's crucial that the baby is born within twenty-four hours of your water breaking, to minimize the complications that can arise in newborns—some of which include meningitis, loss of sight or hearing, and kidney damage.

If this is a subsequent pregnancy for you, the medical community says once GBS positive, always treat as if you were, which means a standard course of antibiotics. However, you may want to consider evaluating this option against what's actually happening (read: insist on test for GBS).

Signs of Labor

Baby Dropping

"Dropping"—one sign that your body is preparing for birth—means that the baby is settling into your pelvis and her head is most likely engaging with your cervix, in preparation for the trip through the birth canal. You may notice that you have a little more room to breathe now! So, take a few breaths as you prepare for birth. Baby is coming soon.

Mucus Plug

The mucus plug is a layer of mucus that blocks the cervix and protects against bacteria entering the uterus throughout your pregnancy. When your cervix begins to dilate to prepare for birth, the mucus plug is discharged. It can be clear, pink, greenish, or slightly bloody, and means that you're on your way toward labor—eventually (it might still be days away). Don't be discouraged if you lose your mucus plug but nothing happens immediately. Some women don't even notice the passing of their mucus plug. If you do notice that you have passed your mucus plug prior to the thirty-seven-week mark, check with your provider to troubleshoot any warning signs of preterm labor.

Braxton-Hicks and Labor Contractions

(See Differentiating Between Braxton-Hicks and Labor Contractions in month eight.)

Effacement

Effacement—often called "cervical ripening" or "cervical thinning"—happens as you get closer to the delivery time. The baby engages with the pelvis, and the cervix (which connects the uterus to the vaginal canal) begins to soften and shorten. Throughout your pregnancy, the cervix is about two to three centimeters; by close to birth, it will be about one centimeter (aka 50 percent effaced). Eventually, when your cervix is 100 percent effaced, it will start to open and you will give birth—simple!

Cervical Dilation

When the cervix begins to open, it's called *dilation*. Typical cervical dilation and labor follows this pattern:

- Latent phase: 0 to 3 centimeters
- Active labor: 4 to 7 centimeters
- Transition: 8 to 10 centimeters
- Complete or ready for birth: 10 centimeters

Water Breaking

You'll most likely know if your water has broken, but to give you a sense, it can be a trickling or a large gush of fluids—as if you've wet yourself, which you have, just not in "that" way. During pregnancy, it isn't uncommon to have some urinary incontinence, especially from anything that causes a down-bearing pressure, like coughing or laughing, but urine has more of an ammonia smell than when your water breaks.

You are more susceptible to infection while you are pregnant, so never use a tampon to contain fluid. If you suspect that your water may have broken during intercourse, *do not introduce anything else* into the vagina at this point, in order to prevent infection.

By the way, if you're reading this right now, and this has already happened, I am wishing you well, as you are about to deliver your baby!

A Note on Baby's Size

Barring any of the positional changes that we discussed in the last chapter, or health concerns that may lead to certain proportional changes in baby, I've rarely seen a woman whose birth canal can't accommodate the size of her baby. Many women get nervous about birthing a large baby, but in the throes of labor, there's really no difference between a couple of pounds. Just remember, it's not the size of your visible hips that matter; your pelvic outlet opens as much as baby needs it to. So, if you're aiming for vaginal birth, go for it. There are always options along the way to assist you in the ultimate goal—a healthy and safe delivery for you and baby.

Herpes Syndrome and Relevance to Birth

Herpes, specifically herpes simplex virus type 2 (HSV-2), is one of the most common sexually transmitted infections. If you have it, it's important to monitor it with your healthcare provider throughout your pregnancy—especially as you near birth, which is the most likely time the virus can potentially be transmitted to the baby.

You can draw on an ancient Egyptian lore: propolis. If you're having an outbreak, some clinical research shows that applying a propolis ointment (see resource section for a recommended brand) significantly improves healing of recurrent genital lesions caused by HSV-2 and may even help heal lesions faster than the acyclovir ointment (a prescription antiviral medication).

A side note: Pemphigoid gestationis (PG) is a rare autoimmune disorder of pregnancy. It was originally named *herpes gestationis* because of the similarity of the blisters, but this condition is not related to herpes virus infection and is usually treated with corticosteroids.

If you have a history of recurrent genital herpes, you may want to consider opting for an oral antiviral medication from thirty-six weeks on as a preventative measure, but if there's no visible outbreak around delivery time, the risk of your baby contracting the virus is less than 1 percent. If you do have an active outbreak or impending symptoms such as tingling, burning, or pain, this could warrant a C-section. Always discuss the nuances of herpes and the health care considerations and treatment options with your provider.

By the way, even cold sores on one's mouth can be dangerous to a newborn. So, be sure you (and anyone your baby comes into contact with) are aware of this. Cold sores can benefit from the same propolis-based ointment noted above (apply five times daily at the start of symptoms).

Cytomegalovirus

Cytomegalovirus is in the same family as herpes, a name which literally means "to creep," a reference to this family of viruses being latent until provoked by things such as stress, fatigue, or exposure to someone else with the virus. It is shared through fluids such as saliva and urine. So, this is mostly an issue after baby is born, and although it is recognized as the leading infectious cause of some congenital issues such as hearing, vision, and brain damage, most babies who are born with cytomegalovirus never develop symptoms or complications. There are no readily available Western treatments, so again we turn to the age-old remedies of boosting up our immunity and, of course, hygiene.

Checklist for Month Nine

- Ready your home to receive you and baby after birth, including stocking freezer with premade food.
- Pack hospital bag.
- Prepare sitz bath ingredients (see month ten).
- Coordinate for placental encapsulation if you're opting for this (see more on this topic in month ten).
- Have your baby!

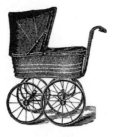

....

Month Ten

"The Golden Month," or the Aftermath

In Chinese medicine, the month after baby is born is still considered an intimate extension of your pregnancy. It is easy for everyone around you to focus primarily on the new baby during this time, and although that may be a welcome aspect of your support, in order for baby to best be taken care of right now, *you* need to be the focus of care and nurturing. A healthy mom is fundamental for a healthy baby—after all, baby benefits from your resources. This postpartum period should emphasize nourishing and replenishing *you*, and by extension, baby will be getting all the nourishment he needs.

The main lifestyle focus for you should be rest and bonding with your infant and incorporating nutritious food, such as a daily dose of the Boosted-Up Chicken Stock (recipe on page 46), for your recovery and continued stamina.

Breastfeeding

There are plenty of conflicting strategies and opinions about how to breastfeed—timed feeding versus feeding-on-demand, for instance—but remember that, just as you know your own body, you will get to know your baby's needs better than anyone. Utilize strategies in conjunction with intuition and experimentation to discover what will work best for you and baby.

That said, breastfeeding is not necessarily as intuitive as it is made out to be. It can be a skill that you learn and develop. Different techniques, combined with persistence and patience, can make a big difference in successful breastfeeding.

By the way, breastfeeding can be a great remedy for postpartum depression. It helps balance hormone swings and increases endorphin levels—but it can also pose some challenges.

There are also some nifty gadgets such as breast pumps (I highly recommend renting or buying a hospital-grade one), nipple shields (very useful if you have small or inverted nipples), and supplemental nursing systems, or SNS, which are tiny tubes that you tape parallel to your nipple to distribute formula. Some women use these to supplement while waiting for the milk supply to kick in. That way, the baby is in training to associate where food comes from and is practicing her latch right from the start. Supply and demand usually start to match up after a while! Don't hesitate to seek out a lactation consultant for more tips.

Here are some strategies to facilitate ease in your experience.

Milk Supply

GENERAL TIPS TO BUILD MILK PRODUCTION

- Decrease your level of stress (the more relaxed you are, the greater the release of prolactin and oxytocin, which facilitates milk production and bonding).
- Stay hydrated with water, stocks, soups, and noncaffeinated teas.

EMPHASIZE THE FOLLOWING FOODS

- Fermented foods (such as miso soup and sauerkraut) in small amounts with each meal
- Soaked oat and barley congee (1 cup grain to 8 cups water, boiled and simmered until porridge-like)
- Beets, carrots, winter squash
- Almonds
- Avocados
- Leafy greens
- Sea vegetables

....

MILK-PRODUCTION TEA

Directions

Boil ½ cup barley in 3 cups of water for twenty-five minutes. Pour into cup and add 1 teaspoon of fennel seeds. Cover and let steep for ten minutes. Optional to also sweeten with honey.

Drink daily as needed.

....

Engorgement

Engorgement, or intense swelling of the breasts, often occurs when milk first comes in, or when baby decides to not take much milk during a feeding. It may be incredibly uncomfortable, but will generally resolve as supply adjusts to baby's demand. To help this adjustment along, apply warmth and gently massage breasts toward the nipples, hand-express the milk to start it flowing, and then encourage baby to nurse.

ADDITIONAL TIPS FOR ENGORGEMENT:

- Soak cabbage or comfrey leaves in cold water and apply to breasts for twenty minutes.
- A hot ginger compress can help when applied under the arms and to the outer areas of the breasts (but not the nipples). Chop up a handful of fresh ginger root, tie it in a muslin bag, and simmer for ten minutes in boiling water. Let it cool just until you can tolerate the temperature on your skin, then lightly squeeze out excess water and apply for five to ten minutes to each spot.

Cracked Nipples

To remedy cracked nipples:

- Check baby's latch.
- Apply vitamin E, aloe vera, or lanolin and ice to nipples in between nursing sessions. (Be sure to clean off the goop before nursing.)
- Express a few drops of milk and rub it into the areola to help the healing time.
- Exposure to sunlight can also be beneficial.

Raw and inflamed breasts can leave you susceptible to infection, so if you develop any flu symptoms, call your provider right away.

Mastitis

Mastitis is an infection that most often originates from engorgement. You can identify it by a reddening of your breasts that can include lumps or streaky areas and may be combined with a fever.

Because mastitis is caused by residual pooling of milk inside the breasts—a fertile ground for bacteria to enter the nipple—the best way to prevent it is to express at each feeding until the milk is gone. Attention to cleanliness, positioning, proper latch, and relaxed nursing on demand can also all help to prevent mastitis. For severe or persistent mastitis, antibiotics may be necessary to prevent abscesses.

Urinary Incontinence after Birth

If you're not already doing kegels regularly, revisit the section on incontinence on page 152. And on a practical note, wearing a pad may be warranted for a while.

A sitz bath with astringent herbs can also help retain some of the leakage and temporarily tighten the muscles while you do the structural rebuilding. It's also a warm and gentle encouragement for healing after birth.

Processing the Placenta

Postpartum Placental Consumption

Many cultures have rituals around disposal or consumption of the placenta. Some traditions include burying the placenta and planting a tree with it that can grow alongside the child. In Chinese medicine, the placenta is traditionally dried and prepared as capsules for the new mother to consume to help her recovery by replenishing her "essence."

This may seem like cannibalism, but many animals "clean up" after their young, and if you're interested in placenta encapsulation, there are folks such as doulas, midwives, and Chinese medicine practitioners who are qualified to safely prepare the dehydrated capsules for you to help you recover and rebuild from birth. However, it should be noted that in some women,

....

POSTPARTUM SITZ BATH

Ingredients

 1 cup Epsom salts

 2 ounces witch hazel

 2 ounces dried calendula

 2 ounces dried chamomile

 2 ounces dried comfrey

 2 ounces dried lavender blossoms

 2 ounces dried lemon balm leaf

 2 ounces dried plantain leaf

 2 ounces dried yarrow

Directions

Combine all ingredients and fill several muslin bags with a handful of the concoction in each bag. To use, fill sitz bath tub (a plastic bin that fits on the toilet seat) with hot water and place one muslin bag into the bath to steep. When the water temperature is tolerable for you, soak for fifteen to twenty minutes.

See the resource section for where to order dried herbs.

....

consuming the placenta can interfere with breastfeeding. So, if you're having any issues with that, discontinue use of your placenta capsules for a few weeks.

Benefits of Placenta Consumption

A trove of research has analyzed the components of the placenta and the potential benefits to its consumption by new moms. Some of the highlights of what the placenta contains and what its benefits are:

- Oxytocin: helps with pain and increases emotional bonding with baby
- Thyroid-stimulating hormone: boosts energy and helps recovery from stressful events

- Interferon: stimulates the immune system to protect against infections
- Gammaglobulin: boosts the immune system and helps protect against postpartum infections
- Prolactin: helps with lactation
- Iron and protein: to reintroduce essential nutrients back into your system to promote healing and recovery

Postpartum Nutrition

Being a new full-time mom is not easy. In order to support you and your little one, you must eat! When you're breastfeeding, you need 300 to 500 more calories per day than you did before you were pregnant. If you're at a loss for what to eat, seek out a local nutrition counselor and enlist your friends and family in a food rotation.

General guidelines for postpartum nutrition include eating easy-to-digest, protein-rich food, eating regularly, and avoiding any food that you notice your baby is sensitive to. Here are some recipes to consider.

....

BONE STOCK WITH POST-PARTUM HERBS

Traditional Chinese Medicine guides mothers to eat certain foods and herbs for the first month after birth to aid recovery. Bone stock is a great way to nourish you and your baby and draw on the ancient Chinese secret of postpartum vitality. So, keep going with or revisit your Boosted-Up Chicken Stock (see recipe page 46) with the addition of the following ingredients added into the cooking process: a palmful of both goji berries and Chinese red dates (also called Jujube).

....

....

YAM, GINGER, AND ADZUKI CONGEE

This is a gentle, nutrient-rich porridge to promote postpartum recovery and give you the protein boost you need for producing breast milk.

Ingredients

> 1 cup white rice
>
> ¼ cup adzuki beans
>
> 1 yam, peeled and coarsely chopped
>
> About an inch of fresh ginger root, chopped
>
> 10 cups water

Directions

Simply place everything in a stock pot or slow cooker and simmer until porridge consistency (approximately four to six hours).

....

BLOOD ORANGE SHRUB

This refreshing, vinegar-based beverage can help consolidate and rebuild fluids that were lost during birth.

Ingredients

> 1 cup freshly squeezed blood orange juice (you can also substitute other citrus if you can't find blood oranges, which tend to be in season from December through May)
>
> 1 cup organic sugar
>
> 1 cup apple cider vinegar
>
> Sparkling water

Directions

Stir the sugar into the blood orange juice, then let sit until the sugar is completely dissolved (1-2 hours). Mix in apple cider vinegar. Add 1 tablespoon to a full cup of sparkling water (to taste) and enjoy.

....

. . . .

MILK-BOOSTING TEA AND COOKIES

The ingredients in the tea, and many of the ingredients in the cookies, are galactagogues (foods that can help increase lactation), while replenishing minerals too.

Tea Ingredients

¼ cup dried alfalfa

½ cup fennel seeds

¼ cup dried nettle

½ cup dried red raspberry leaves

¼ cup dried dandelion leaves

1 cinnamon stick

3 cloves

Tea Directions

Combine all of the ingredients together in a large jar and shake to blend. Fill a tea ball with a tablespoon or two of the blend and place in a cup of boiled water. Let infuse for about ten minutes. Add a touch of organic, whole cream, or homemade almond milk (see recipe page 32 if you'd like).

Cookie Ingredients

2 cups organic rolled oats

1 tablespoon freshly ground fennel seeds

2 tablespoons freshly ground flax seeds

½ cup organic coconut sugar

¼ cup tapioca flour

¼ cup nutritional yeast flakes

1 teaspoon aluminum-free baking powder

½ teaspoon baking soda

½ teaspoon sea salt

1 teaspoon cinnamon

½ cup almond butter or tahini

¼ cup plus 2 tablespoons coconut oil, melted, plus extra for pan

2 tablespoons molasses

2 eggs

½ teaspoon organic almond extract

Cookie Directions

Pre-heat oven to 350 degrees Fahrenheit. Grease a cookie sheet with coconut oil. Place oats into a high-speed blender or food processor and blend until coarsely powdered. Grind fennel and flax seeds in a coffee grinder or with a mortar and pestle until powdered. Combine all dry ingredients into a bowl and mix together. In a separate bowl, combine almond or tahini butter, melted coconut oil, molasses, eggs, and almond extract. Stir well. Pour the wet ingredients into the dry ingredients. Mix with a spoon or hands. Form small balls and gently flatten with back of spoon. Bake for fifteen to twenty minutes or until slightly brown. Remove from oven and transfer cookies to a cooling rack. Store in an airtight glass container. Enjoy a cookie with your tea daily!

General Postpartum Support Tips

Get Sleep

I can't say enough about how great a postpartum doula is for the first week. If you can get a little sleep, your overall coping skills and bonding ability will probably improve greatly.

Receive Massage

Nurturing touch can be very replenishing after birth. See if you can find someone who can come to your house.

Navigate Mood

It's normal to feel overtaxed. Just keep an eye on it and make sure it doesn't get incapacitating. You can enlist a therapist or a psychiatrist to give you support and help you assess the possible need for breastfeeding-safe medication.

Tell Your Story

Find a forum, either in person or online, to share your birth story. This can be a very therapeutic way to process your experience.

The Aftermath

Now that you've concluded your pregnancy journey, the support you need is just beginning. Keep drawing on all the ways you've learned to care for during your pregnancy, and don't hesitate to seek out resources during your post-partum period, or as I call it, the aftermath.

·····························

Resources

All herbal products mentioned throughout the book can be found at:
www.mountainroseherbs.com

PRENATAL VITAMINS

www.rainbowlight.com/prenatal-vitamins-prenatal-one
-multivitamin.aspx

BABY FORMULA

HIPP (a formula produced in England that can be procured from varying
online sources)

YIN-CARE HERBAL WASH

www.yincare.com

SEEDED PAPER FOR BABY ANNOUNCEMENTS

www.botanicalpaperworks.com

PROPOLIS OINTMENT

www.herstat.com

GUIDED IMAGERY

www.thehealingmind.org

PREGNANCY-SAFE TINCTURES

www.wishgardenherbs.com

BOOK RECOMMENDATIONS

Ina May's Guide to Childbirth by Ina May Gaskin

The Thinking Woman's Guide to a Better Birth by Henci Goer and Rhonda Wheeler

The Birth Book: Everything You Need to Know to Have a Safe and Satisfying Birth by William Sears

Gentle Birth Choices by Barbara Harper

The Birth Partner by Penny Simkin

Bibliography

Ablove, Robert H., and Tova S. Ablove. "Prevalence of Carpal Tunnel Syndrome in Pregnant Women." *WMJ* 108 (July 2009): 194–6. http://www.ncbi.nlm.nih.gov/pubmed/19753825.

Abramowicz, J. S., F. W. Kremkau, and E. Merz. "Obstetrical Ultrasound: Can the Fetus Hear the Wave and Feel the Heat?" *Ultraschall in der Medizin* 33 (June 2012): 215–7. http://www.ncbi.nlm.nih.gov/pubmed/22700164.

Acar, H. Volkan. "Acupuncture Points in the Book of Şerefeddin Sabuncuoğlu, a 15th Century Turkish Physician." *Acupuncture in Medicine: Journal of the British Medical Acupuncture Society* 33 (February 2015): 72–6. http://www.ncbi.nlm.nih.gov/pubmed/25380833.

ACOG. "Ethical Issues in Genetic Testing." http://www.acog.org/Resources-And-Publications/Committee-Opinions/Committee-on-Ethics/Ethical-Issues-in-Genetic-Testing.

Adam, Margaret P., Janine E. Polifka, and J. M. Friedman. "Evolving Knowledge of the Teratogenicity of Medications in Human Pregnancy." *American Journal of Medical Genetics. Part C, Seminars in Medical Genetics* 157C (August 2011): 175–82. http://www.ncbi.nlm.nih.gov/pubmed/21766440.

Aditi, Anupam, and David Y. Graham. "Vitamin C, Gastritis, and Gastric Disease: A Historical Review and Update." *Digestive Diseases and Sciences* 57 (October 2012): 2504–15. http://www.pubmedcentral.nih.gov

/articlerender.fcgi?artid=3874117&tool=pmcentrez&
rendertype=abstract.

Adler, Ben, and Alejandro de la Pena Moctezuma. "Leptospira and Leptospirosis." *Veterinary Microbiology* 140 (January 2010): 287–96. http://
www.ncbi.nlm.nih.gov/pubmed/19345023.

Adukauskiene, Dalia, Venta Vizgirdaite, Kestutis Rimaitis, and Asta
Aliuskeviciene. "Hemolysis, Elevated Liver Enzymes, and Low Platelet Count Syndrome." *Medicina* 42 (Kaunas, Lithuania, January 2006):
695–702. http://www.ncbi.nlm.nih.gov/pubmed/17028466.

Alamillo, Christina M. L., Morris Fiddler, and Eugene Pergament.
"Increased Nuchal Translucency in the Presence of Normal Chromo-
somes: What's Next?" *Current Opinion in Obstetrics & Gynecology* 24
(March 2012): 102–8. http://www.ncbi.nlm.nih.gov/pubmed/22277886.

Aldridge, A., J. V. Aranda, and A. H. Neims. "Caffeine Metabolism in the
Newborn." *Clinical Pharmacology and Therapeutics* 25 (April 1979):
447–53. http://www.ncbi.nlm.nih.gov/pubmed/428190.

Alfarra, Helmi Y., Sabreen R. Alfarra, and Mai F. Sadiq. "Neural Tube
Defects Between Folate Metabolism and Genetics." *Indian Journal of
Human Genetics* 17 (September 2011): 126–31. http://www
.pubmedcentral.nih.gov/articlerender.fcgi?artid=3276979&tool=
pmcentrez&rendertype=abstract.

Alfirevic, Z., K. Sundberg, and S. Brigham. "Amniocentesis and Chorionic
Villus Sampling for Prenatal Diagnosis." *The Cochrane Database of Systematic Reviews* (September 1996): CD003252. http://www
.pubmedcentral.nih.gov/articlerender.fcgi?artid=4171981&tool=
pmcentrez&rendertype=abstract.

Algul, Ayhan, Cengiz Basoglu, Mehmet Z. Kiralp, and Levent Ozcakar.
"Fibromyalgia in Between: Where Do the Musculoskeletal Physicians
and Psychiatrists Stand?" *Acta Reumatológica Portuguesa* 33, no. 4:
477–8. http://www.ncbi.nlm.nih.gov/pubmed/19107094.

Alldred, S. Kate, Jonathan J. Deeks, Boliang Guo, James P. Neilson, and
Zarko Alfirevic. "Second Trimester Serum Tests for Down's Syndrome
Screening." *The Cochrane Database of Systematic Reviews* 6 (January
2012): CD009925. http://www.ncbi.nlm.nih.gov/pubmed/22696388.

Allen, Peggy Rosati. "Chronic Fatigue Syndrome: Implications for Women
and Their Health Care Providers During the Childbearing Years."

Journal of Midwifery & Women's Health 53 (July–August 2008): 289–301; quiz 399. http://www.ncbi.nlm.nih.gov/pubmed/18586181.

Al-Sereiti, M. R., K. M. Abu-Amer, and P. Sen. "Pharmacology of Rosemary (Rosmarinus officinalis Linn.) and Its Therapeutic Potentials." *Indian Journal of Experimental Biology* 37 (February 1999): 124–30. http://www.ncbi.nlm.nih.gov/pubmed/10641130.

Alwan, Sura, and A. Dessa Sadovnick. "Multiple Sclerosis and Pregnancy: Maternal Considerations." *Women's Health* (July 2012): 399–414. http://www.ncbi.nlm.nih.gov/pubmed/22757731.

Alwan, S., I. M. Yee, M. Dybalski, C. Guimond, E. Dwosh, T. M. Greenwood, R. Butler, and A. D. Sadovnick. "Reproductive Decision Making After the Diagnosis of Multiple Sclerosis (MS)." *Multiple Sclerosis* 19 (March 2013): 351–8. http://www.ncbi.nlm.nih.gov/pubmed/22760102.

Andrade, Susan E., Jerry H. Gurwitz, Robert L. Davis, K. Arnold Chan, Jonathan A. Finkelstein, Kris Fortman, Heather McPhillips, Marsha A. Raebel, Douglas Roblin, David H. Smith, Marianne Ulcickas Yood, Abraham N. Morse, and Richard Platt. "Prescription Drug Use in Pregnancy." *American Journal of Obstetrics and Gynecology* 191 (August 2004): 398–407. http://www.ncbi.nlm.nih.gov/pubmed/15343213.

Andrews, C. M., and L. M. O'Neill. "Use of Pelvic Tilt Exercise for Ligament Pain Relief." *Journal of Nurse-Midwifery* 39 (December 1994): 370–4. http://ovidsp.ovid.com/ovidweb.

Aractingi, S., N. Berkane, P. Bertheau, C. Le Goue, J. Dausset, S. Uzan, and E. D. Carosella. "Fetal DNA in Skin of Polymorphic Eruptions of Pregnancy." *Lancet* 352 (December 1998): 1898–901. http://www.ncbi.nlm.nih.gov/pubmed/9863788.

Aronson, I. K., S. Bond, V. C. Fiedler, S. Vomvouras, D. Gruber, and C. Ruiz. "Pruritic Urticarial Papules and Plaques of Pregnancy: Clinical and Immunopathologic Observations in 57 Patients." *Journal of the American Academy of Dermatology* 39 (December 1998): 933–9. http://www.ncbi.nlm.nih.gov/pubmed/9843004.

Bacq, Yannick. "Liver Diseases Unique to Pregnancy: A 2010 Update." *Clinics and Research in Hepatology and Gastroenterology* 35 (March 2011): 182–93. http://www.ncbi.nlm.nih.gov/pubmed/21310683.

Bagshaw, M. "Pregnancy and In-Flight Cosmic Radiation." *Aviation, Space, and Environmental Medicine* 70 (May 1999): 533. http://www.ncbi .nlm.nih.gov/pubmed/10332954.

Bankova, V., A. S. Galabov, D. Antonova, N. Vilhelmova, and B. Di Perri. "Chemical Composition of Propolis Extract ACF® and Activity Against Herpes Simplex Virus." *Phytomedicine: International Journal of Phytotherapy and Phytopharmacology* 21 (September 2013): 1432–8. http:// www.ncbi.nlm.nih.gov/pubmed/25022206.

Barger, Mary K. "Maternal Nutrition and Perinatal Outcomes." *Journal of Midwifery & Women's Health* 55 (November–December 2010): 502–11. http://www.ncbi.nlm.nih.gov/pubmed/20974412.

Barish, Robert J. "In-Flight Radiation Exposure During Pregnancy." *Obstetrics and Gynecology* 103 (June 2004): 1326–30. http://www.ncbi .nlm.nih.gov/pubmed/15172873.

Barouei, J., M. C. Adams, and D. M. Hodgson. "Prophylactic Role of Maternal Administration of Probiotics in the Prevention of Irritable Bowel Syndrome." *Medical Hypotheses* 73 (November 2009): 764–7. http:// www.ncbi.nlm.nih.gov/pubmed/19481357.

Beard, M. P., and G. W. M. Millington. "Recent Developments in the Specific Dermatoses of Pregnancy." *Clinical and Experimental Dermatology* 37 (January 2012): 1–4; quiz 5. http://www.ncbi.nlm.nih.gov /pubmed/22007708.

Beauchamp, Gary K., and Julie A. Mennella. "Flavor Perception in Human Infants: Development and Functional Significance." *Digestion* 83, (March 2011): 1–6. http://www.pubmedcentral.nih.gov/articlerender .fcgi?artid=3202923&tool=pmcentrez&rendertype=abstract.

Bikov, Andras, Renata Bocskei, Noemi Eszes, Aniko Bohacs, Gyorgy Losonczy, Janos Rigo, Ildiko Horvath, and Lilla Tamasi. "Circulating Survivin Levels in Healthy and Asthmatic Pregnancy." *Reproductive Biology and Endocrinology* 12 (January 2014): 93. http://www .pubmedcentral.nih.gov/articlerender.fcgi?artid=4189549&tool= pmcentrez&rendertype=abstract.

Bisset, L. R., T. M. Fiddes, W. R. Gillett, P. D. Wilson, and J. F. Griffin. "Altered Humoral Immunoregulation During Human Pregnancy." *American Journal of Reproductive Immunology* 23 (May 1990): 4–9. http:// www.ncbi.nlm.nih.gov/pubmed/2397041.

Blanquisett, Abraham Hernández, Carmen Herrero Vicent, Joaquín Gavilá Gregori, Ángel Guerrero Zotano, Vicente Guillem Porta, and Amparo Ruiz Simón. "Breast Cancer in Pregnancy: An Institutional Experience." *Ecancermedicalscience* 9 (January 2015): 551. http://www .pubmedcentral.nih.gov/articlerender.fcgi?artid=4531131&tool= pmcentrez&rendertype=abstract.

Bloom, Erica, Eva Nyman, Aime Must, Christina Pehrson, and Lennart Larsson. "Molds and Mycotoxins in Indoor Environments: A Survey in Water-Damaged Buildings." *Journal of Occupational and Environmental Hygiene* 6 (October 2009): 671–8. http://www.ncbi.nlm .nih.gov/pubmed/19757292.

Boivin, Jacky, and Deborah Lancastle. "Medical Waiting Periods: Imminence, Emotions and Coping." *Women's Health* 6 (London, January 2010): 59–69. http://www.ncbi.nlm.nih.gov/pubmed/20088730.

Bonapace, E. S., and R. S. Fisher. "Constipation and Diarrhea in Pregnancy." *Gastroenterology Clinics of North America* 27 (March 1998): 197–211. http://www.ncbi.nlm.nih.gov/pubmed/9546090.

Boskey, E. R., R. A. Cone, K. J. Whaley, and T. R. Moench. "Origins of Vaginal Acidity: High D/L Lactate Ratio Is Consistent with Bacteria Being the Primary Source." *Human Reproduction* 16 (September 2001): 1809–13. http://www.ncbi.nlm.nih.gov/pubmed/11527880.

Brent, R. L. "The Effects of Embryonic and Fetal Exposure to X-ray, Microwaves, and Ultrasound." *Clinics in Perinatology* 13 (September 1986): 615–48. http://www.ncbi.nlm.nih.gov/pubmed/3533368.

Brisinda, G. "How to Treat Haemorrhoids. Prevention Is Best; Haemorrhoidectomy Needs Skilled Operators. *BMJ: British Medical Journal* 321 (September 9, 2000): 582–3. http://www.pubmedcentral.nih .gov/articlerender.fcgi?artid=1118483&tool=pmcentrez& rendertype=abstract.

Brocklehurst, P., and R. French. "The Association Between Maternal HIV Infection and Perinatal Outcome: A Systematic Review of the Literature and Meta-Analysis." *British Journal of Obstetrics and Gynaecology* 105 (August 1998): 836–48. http://www.ncbi.nlm.nih .gov/pubmed/9746375.

Brocklehurst, P., and J. Volmink. "Antiretrovirals for Reducing the Risk of Mother-to-Child Transmission of HIV Infection." *The Cochrane*

Database of Systematic Reviews (January 2002): CD003510. http://www.ncbi.nlm.nih.gov/pubmed/12076484.

Brown, Zane. "Preventing Herpes Simplex Virus Transmission to the Neonate." *Herpes: The Journal of the IHMF* 11, Suppl 3 (August 2004): 175A–186A. http://www.ncbi.nlm.nih.gov/pubmed/15319088.

Bzowej, Natalie H. "Optimal Management of the Hepatitis B Patient Who Desires Pregnancy or Is Pregnant." *Current Hepatitis Reports* 11 (June 2012): 82–9. http://www.pubmedcentral.nih.gov/articlerender.fcgi?artid=3364416&tool=pmcentrez&rendertype=abstract.

Camargo, Antonio, Juan Ruano, Juan M. Fernandez, Laurence D. Parnell, Anabel Jimenez, Monica Santos-Gonzalez, Carmen Marin, Pablo Perez-Martinez, Marino Uceda, Jose Lopez-Miranda, and Francisco Perez-Jimenez. "Gene Expression Changes in Mononuclear Cells in Patients with Metabolic Syndrome After Acute Intake of Phenol-Rich Virgin Olive Oil." *BMC Genomics* 11 (January 2010): 253. http://www.pubmedcentral.nih.gov/articlerender.fcgi?artid=2874810&tool=pmcentrez&rendertype=abstract.

Camilleri, Michael. "Probiotics and Irritable Bowel Syndrome: Rationale, Putative Mechanisms, and Evidence of Clinical Efficacy." *Journal of Clinical Gastroenterology* 40 (March 2006): 264–9. http://www.ncbi.nlm.nih.gov/pubmed/16633134.

Casey, Brian M., and Susan M. Cox. "Cholecystitis in Pregnancy." *Infectious Diseases in Obstetrics and Gynecology* 4 (January 1996): 303–9. http://www.pubmedcentral.nih.gov/articlerender.fcgi?artid=2364506&tool=pmcentrez&rendertype=abstract.

Catalano, P. M., N. M. Roman-Drago, S. B. Amini, and E. A. Sims. "Longitudinal Changes in Body Composition and Energy Balance in Lean Women with Normal and Abnormal Glucose Tolerance During Pregnancy." *American Journal of Obstetrics and Gynecology* 179 (July 1998): 156–65. http://www.ncbi.nlm.nih.gov/pubmed/9704782.

Chang, Anne Lynn S., Yolanda Z. Agredano, and Alexa Boer Kimball. "Risk Factors Associated with Striae Gravidarum." *Journal of the American Academy of Dermatology* 51 (December 2004): 881–5. http://www.ncbi.nlm.nih.gov/pubmed/15583577.

Chen, Kai, Ugochi Akoma, Andrea Anderson, Heather Mertz, and Michael D. Quartermain. "Prenatally Diagnosed Single Umbilical Artery: The

Role and Relationship of Additional Risk Factors in the Fetus for Congenital Heart Disease." *Journal of Clinical Ultrasound* 44 (February 2016): 113–7. http://www.ncbi.nlm.nih.gov/pubmed/26178181.

Chen, Morie M., Fergus V. Coakley, Anjali Kaimal, and Russell K. Laros. "Guidelines for Computed Tomography and Magnetic Resonance Imaging Use During Pregnancy and Lactation. *Obstetrics and Gynecology* 112 (August 2008): 333–40. http://www.ncbi.nlm.nih.gov/pubmed/18669732.

Chibber, Rachana, M. Hisham Al-Sibai, and Noura Qahtani. "Adverse Outcome of Pregnancy Following Air Travel: A Myth or a Concern?" *The Australian & New Zealand Journal of Obstetrics & Gynaecology* 46 (February2006): 24–8. http://www.ncbi.nlm.nih.gov/pubmed/16441688.

Chorostowska-Wynimko, J., E. Skopińska-Rozewska, E. Sommer, E. Rogala, P. Skopiński, and E. Wojtasik. "Multiple Effects of Theobromine on Fetus Development and Postnatal Status of the Immune System." *International Journal of Tissue Reactions* 26 (January 2004): 53–60. http://www.ncbi.nlm.nih.gov/pubmed/15573693.

Cohen, Taylor Sitarik, and Alice Prince. "Cystic Fibrosis: A Mucosal Immunodeficiency Syndrome." *Nature Medicine* 18 (April 2012): 509–19. http://www.pubmedcentral.nih.gov/articlerender.fcgi?artid=3577071&tool=pmcentrez&rendertype=abstract.

Cooper, Marvin C. "The Pregnant Traveller." *Travel Medicine and Infectious Disease* 4 (May–July 2006): 196–201. http://www.ncbi.nlm.nih.gov/pubmed/16887741.

Corrado, F., R. D'Anna, G. Di Vieste, D. Giordano, B. Pintaudi, A. Santamaria, and A. Di Benedetto. "The Effect of Myoinositol Supplementation on Insulin Resistance in Patients with Gestational Diabetes." *Diabetic Medicine* 28 (August 2011): 972–5. http://www.ncbi.nlm.nih.gov/pubmed/21414183.

Costigan, Kathleen A., Heather L. Sipsma, and Janet A. DiPietro. "Pregnancy Folklore Revisited: The Case of Heartburn and Hair." *Birth* 33 (December 2006): 311–4. http://www.ncbi.nlm.nih.gov/pubmed/17150070.

Cox, T. E., L. D. Smythe, and L. K. Leung. "Flying Foxes as Carriers of Pathogenic Leptospira Species." *Journal of Wildlife Diseases* 41 (October 2005): 753–7. http://www.ncbi.nlm.nih.gov/pubmed/16456164.

Culpepper, L., and B. Jack. "Psychosocial Issues in Pregnancy." *Primary Care* 20 (September 1993): 599–619. http://www.ncbi.nlm.nih.gov /pubmed/8378453.

Dancey, Anne, M. Khan, J. Dawson, and F. Peart. "Gigantomastia: A Classi-fication and Review of the Literature." *Journal of Plastic, Reconstructive & Aesthetic Surgery* 61 (January 2008): 493–502. http://www .ncbi.nlm.nih.gov/pubmed/18054304.

Demir, Uygar Levent, Bilge Cetinkaya Demir, Ege Oztosun, Ozlem Ozgun Uyaniklar, and Gokhan Ocakoglu. "The Effects of Pregnancy on Nasal Physiology." *International Forum of Allergy & Rhinology* 5 (February 2015): 162–6. http://www.ncbi.nlm.nih.gov/pubmed/25348597.

De-Regil, Luz Maria, Cristina Palacios, Ali Ansary, Regina Kulier, and Juan Pablo Pena-Rosas. "Vitamin D Supplementation for Women During Pregnancy." *The Cochrane Database of Systematic Reviews* 2 (January 2012): CD008873. http://www.pubmedcentral.nih.gov/articlerender .fcgi?artid=3747784&tool=pmcentrez&rendertype=abstract.

Devine, P. C., and F. D. Malone. "First Trimester Screening for Structural Fetal Abnormalities: Nuchal Translucency Sonography." *Seminars in Perinatology* 23 (October 1999): 382–92. http://www.ncbi.nlm.nih .gov/pubmed/10551791.

"Diagnosis and Treatment of Sleep Disorders: A Brief Review for Cli-nicians." *Dialogues in Clinical Neuroscience* 5 (December 2003): 371–88. http://www.pubmedcentral.nih.gov/articlerender .fcgi?artid=3181779&tool=pmcentrez&rendertype=abstract.

"Dietary Allowances and Intakes During Pregnancy." http://www .perinatology.com/Reference/RDApregnancy.htm.

Di Renzo, Gian Carlo, Eleonora Brillo, Maila Romanelli, Giuseppina Por-caro, Federica Capanna, Tomi T. Kanninen, Sandro Gerli, and Graziano Clerici. "Potential Effects of Chocolate on Human Pregnancy: A Ran-domized Controlled Trial." *The Journal of Maternal-Fetal & Neonatal Medicine* 25 (October 2012): 1860–7. http://www.ncbi.nlm .nih.gov/pubmed/22537244.

Disanto, Giulio, George Chaplin, Julia M. Morahan, Gavin Giovannoni, Elina Hypponen, George C. Ebers, and Sreeram V. Ramagopalan. "Month of Birth, Vitamin D and Risk of Immune-Mediated Disease: A Case Control Study." *BMC Medicine* 10 (January 2012): 69. http://www.

pubmedcentral.nih.gov/articlerender
.fcgi?artid=3395583&tool=pmcentrez&rendertype=abstract.

Dogra, Vikram, Raj Mohan Paspulati, and Shweta Bhatt. "First Trimester Bleeding Evaluation." *Ultrasound Quarterly* 21 (June 2005): 69–85; quiz 149–50, 153–4. http://www.ncbi.nlm.nih.gov/pubmed/15905817.

Dzieciolowska-Baran, Edyta, Iwona Teul-Swiniarska, Aleksandra Gawlikowska-Sroka, Iwona Poziomkowska-Gesicka, and Zbigniew Zietek. "Rhinitis as a Cause of Respiratory Disorders During Pregnancy." *Advances in Experimental Medicine and Biology* 755 (January 2013): 213–20. http://www.ncbi.nlm.nih.gov/pubmed/22826069.

Edenborough, F. P., D. E. Stableforth, A. K. Webb, W. E. Mackenzie, and D. L. Smith. "Outcome of Pregnancy in Women with Cystic Fibrosis." *Thorax* 50 (February 1995): 170–4. http://www.pubmedcentral.nih.gov/articlerender.fcgi?artid=473918&tool=pmcentrez&rendertype=abstract.

Enck, Paul, Ute Martens, and Sibylle Klosterhalfen. "The Psyche and the Gut." *World Journal of Gastroenterology* 13 (July 2007): 3405–8. http://www.pubmedcentral.nih.gov/articlerender.fcgi?artid=4146774&tool=pmcentrez&rendertype=abstract.

Engineer, Leela, Kailash Bhol, and A. Razzaque Ahmed. "Pemphigoid Gestationis: A Review." *American Journal of Obstetrics and Gynecology* 183 (August 2000): 483–491. http://www.ncbi.nlm.nih.gov/pubmed/10942491.

Enzensberger, C., C. Pulvermacher, J. Degenhardt, A. Kawacki, U. Germer, U. Gembruch, M. Krapp, J. Weichert, and R. Axt-Fliedner."Fetal Loss Rate and Associated Risk Factors After Amniocentesis, Chorionic Villus Sampling and Fetal Blood Sampling." *Ultraschall in der Medizin* 33 (December 2012): E75–9. http://www.ncbi.nlm.nih.gov/pubmed/22623130.

Ernst, E. "Herbal Medicinal Products During Pregnancy: Are They Safe?" *BJOG: An International Journal of Obstetrics and Gynaecology* 109 (March 2002): 227–35. http://www.ncbi.nlm.nih.gov/pubmed/11950176.

Facco, Francesca L., Jamie Kramer, Kim H. Ho, Phyllis C. Zee, and William A. Grobman. "Sleep Disturbances in Pregnancy." *Obstetrics and Gynecology* 115 (January 2010): 77–83. http://www.ncbi.nlm.nih.gov/pubmed/20027038.

Falagas, M. E., G. I. Betsi, and S. Athanasiou. "Probiotics for the Treatment of Women with Bacterial Vaginosis." *Clinical Microbiology and Infection: The Official Publication of the European Society of Clinical Microbiology and Infectious Diseases* 13 (July 2007): 657–64. http://www .ncbi.nlm.nih.gov/pubmed/17633390.

Fantz, C. R., S. Dagogo-Jack, J. H. Ladenson, and A. M. Gronowski. "Thyroid Function During Pregnancy." *Clinical Chemistry* 45 (December 1999): 2250–8. http://www.ncbi.nlm.nih.gov/pubmed/10585360.

Fazzari, Marco, Andres Trostchansky, Francisco J. Schopfer, Sonia R. Salvatore, Beatriz Sanchez-Calvo, Dario Vitturi, Raquel Valderrama, Juan B. Barroso, Rafael Radi, Bruce A. Freeman, and Homero Rubbo. "Olives and Olive Oil Are Sources of Electrophilic Fatty Acid Nitroalkenes." *PloS One* 9 (January 2014): e84884. http://www.pubmedcentral.nih.gov /articlerender .fcgi?artid=3891761&tool=pmcentrez&rendertype= abstract.

Ficarra, Giuseppe, and Catalena Birek. "Oral Herpes Simplex Virus Infection in Pregnancy: What Are the Concerns?" *JCDA: Journal Canadian Dental Association* 75 (September 2009): 523–6. http://www .ncbi.nlm.nih.gov/pubmed/19744363.

Fichera, M. E., and D. S. Roos. "A Plastid Organelle as a Drug Target in Apicomplexan Parasites." *Nature* 390 (November 1997): 407–9. http:// www.ncbi.nlm.nih.gov/pubmed/9389481.

Finkelsztejn, A., and J. B. B. Brooks, F. M. Paschoal, and Y. D. Fragoso. "What Can We Really Tell Women with Multiple Sclerosis Regarding Pregnancy? A Systematic Review and Meta-Analysis of the Literature." *BJOG: An International Journal of Obstetrics and Gynaecology* 118 (June 2011): 790–7. http://www.ncbi.nlm.nih.gov/pubmed/21401856.

Flaxman, S. M. and P. W. Sherman. "Morning Sickness: A Mechanism for Protecting Mother and Embryo." *The Quarterly Review of Biology* 75 (June 2000): 113–48. http://www.ncbi.nlm.nih.gov/pubmed/10858967.

Freeman, Mala, Alessandro Ghidini, Catherine Y. Spong, Nana Tchabo, Patricia Z. Bannon, and John C. Pezzullo. "Does Air Travel Affect Pregnancy Outcome?" *Archives of Gynecology and Obstetrics* 269 (May 2004): 274–7. http://www.ncbi.nlm.nih.gov/pubmed/15205979.

Friedberg, W., K. Copeland, F. E. Duke, K. O'Brien, and E. B. Darden."Radiation Exposure During Air Travel: Guidance Provided by the Federal

Aviation Administration for Air Carrier Crews." *Health Physics* 79 (November 2000): 591–5. http://www.ncbi.nlm.nih.gov /pubmed/11045535.

Gagnon, Alain, R. Douglas Wilson, Franccois Audibert, Victoria M. Allen, Claire Blight, Jo-Ann Brock, Valerie A. Desilets, Jo-Ann Johnson, Sylvie Langlois, Anne Summers, and Philip Wyatt. "Obstetrical Complications Associated with Abnormal Maternal Serum Markers Analytes." *Journal of Obstetrics and Gynaecology Canada* 30 (October 2008): 918–49. http://www.ncbi.nlm.nih.gov/pubmed/19038077.

Galbarczyk, Andrzej. "Unexpected Changes in Maternal Breast Size During Pregnancy in Relation to Infant Sex: An Evolutionary Interpretation." *American Journal of Human Biology* 23 (July 2011): 560–2. http:// www.ncbi.nlm.nih.gov/pubmed/21544894.

Garnica, A. D., and W. Y. Chan. "The Role of the Placenta in Fetal Nutrition and Growth." *Journal of the American College of Nutrition* 15 (June 1996): 206–22. http://www.ncbi.nlm.nih.gov/pubmed/8935436.

Geake, James, Eli Dabscheck, and David Reid. "Hemolysis, Elevated Liver Enzymes, and Low Platelet (HELLP) Syndrome in a 26-Year-Old Woman with Cystic Fibrosis: A Case Report." *Journal of Medical Case Reports* 6 (January 2012): 134. http://www.pubmedcentral.nih.gov/articlerender .fcgi?artid=3416743&tool=pmcentrez&rendertype=abstract.

Geeze, D. S. "Pregnancy and In-Flight Cosmic Radiation." *Aviation, Space, and Environmental Medicine* 69 (November 1998): 1061–4. http:// www.ncbi.nlm.nih.gov/pubmed/9819162.

George, Adekunle Olufemi, Olayiwola Babatunde Shittu, Eokezie Enwerem, Mitchell Wachtel, and Olufemi Kuti. "The Incidence of Lower Mid-Trunk Hyperpigmentation (Linea Nigra) Is Affected by Sex Hormone Levels." *Journal of the National Medical Association* 97 (May 2005): 685–8. http://www.pubmedcentral.nih.gov/articlerender .fcgi?artid=2569341&tool=pmcentrez&rendertype=abstract.

Glantz, Anna, Hanns-Ulrich Marschall, and Lars-Ake Mattsson. "Intrahepatic Cholestasis of Pregnancy: Relationships Between Bile Acid Levels and Fetal Complication Rates." *Hepatology* 40 (August 2004): 467–74. http://www.ncbi.nlm.nih.gov/pubmed/15368452.

Glantz, J. C., and K. E. Kedley. "Concepts and Controversies in the Management of Group B Streptococcus During Pregnancy." *Birth* 25 (March 1998): 45–53. http://www.ncbi.nlm.nih.gov/pubmed/9534505.

Glinoer, D. "What Happens to the Normal Thyroid During Pregnancy?" *Thyroid: Official Journal of the American Thyroid Association* 9 (July 1999): 631–5. http://www.ncbi.nlm.nih.gov/pubmed/10447005.

Glinoer, Daniel. "The Importance of Iodine Nutrition During Pregnancy." *Public Health Nutrition* 10 (December 2007): 1542–6. http://www.ncbi .nlm.nih.gov/pubmed/18053277.

Gluck, Paul A., and Joan C. Gluck. "A Review of Pregnancy Outcomes After Exposure to Orally Inhaled or Intranasal Budesonide." *Current Medical Research and Opinion* 21 (July 2005): 1075–84. http://www.ncbi.nlm. nih.gov/pubmed/16004676.

Gnoth, C., and S. Johnson. "Strips of Hope: Accuracy of Home Pregnancy Tests and New Developments." *Geburtshilfe und Frauenheilkunde* 74 (July 2014): 661–9. http://www.pubmedcentral.nih.gov/articlerender .fcgi?artid=4119102&tool=pmcentrez&rendertype=abstract.

Goetzl, Laura. "Adverse Pregnancy Outcomes After Abnormal First-Trimester Screening for Aneuploidy." *Clinics in Laboratory Medicine* 30 (September 2010): 613–28. http://www.pubmedcentral.nih.gov /articlerender.fcgi?artid=2905811&tool=pmcentrez&rendertype =abstract.

Goldsmith, L. T., G. Weiss, and B. G. Steinetz. "Relaxin and Its Role in Pregnancy." *Endocrinology and Metabolism Clinics of North America* 24 (March 1995): 171–86. http://www.ncbi.nlm.nih.gov/pubmed/7781625.

Gracia, Clarisa R., Mary D. Sammel, Jesse Chittams, Amy C. Hummel, Alka Shaunik, and Kurt T. Barnhart. "Risk Factors for Spontaneous Abortion in Early Symptomatic First-Trimester Pregnancies." *Obstetrics and Gynecology* 106 (November 2005): 993–9. http://www.ncbi.nlm.nih .gov/pubmed/16260517.

Gromnica-Ihle, E., and M. Ostensen. "Pregnancy in Patients with Rheumatoid Arthritis and Inflammatory Spondylarthropathies." *Zeitschrift für Rheumatologie* 65 (May 2006): 209–12, 214–6. http://www.ncbi.nlm .nih.gov/pubmed/16670812.

Grossman, Richard A. "In-Flight Radiation Exposure During Pregnancy." *Obstetrics and Gynecology* 104 (September 2004): 630. http://www.ncbi.nlm.nih.gov/pubmed/15339781.

Gunawardena, Dhanushka, Niloo Karunaweera, Samiuela Lee, Frank van Der Kooy, David G. Harman, Ritesh Raju, Louise Bennett, Erika Gyengesi, Nikolaus J. Sucher, and Gerald Munch. "Anti-inflammatory Activity of Cinnamon (C. Zeylanicum and C. Cassia) Extracts - Identification of E-cinnamaldehyde and O-methoxy Cinnamaldehyde as the Most Potent Bioactive Compounds." *Food & Function* 6 (March 2015): 910–9. http://www.ncbi.nlm.nih.gov/pubmed/25629927.

Gungorduk, K., A. Sahbaz, A. Ozdemir, M. Gokcu, M. Sancı, and M. F. Kose. "Management of Cervical Cancer During Pregnancy." *Journal of Obstetrics and Gynaecology: The Journal of the Institute of Obstetrics and Gynaecology* (October 2015): 1–6. http://www.ncbi.nlm.nih.gov/pubmed/26467977.

Gupta, R., M. Dhyani, T. Kendzerska, S. R. Pandi-Perumal, A. S. BaHammam, P. Srivanitchapoom, S. Pandey, and M. Hallett. "Restless Legs Syndrome and Pregnancy: Prevalence, Possible Pathophysiological Mechanisms and Treatment." *Acta Neurologica Scandinavica* (October 2015). http://www.ncbi.nlm.nih.gov/pubmed/26482928.

Hubner, Astrid, Alexander Krafft, Sonja Gadient, Esther Werth, Roland Zimmermann, and Claudio L. Bassetti. "Characteristics and Determinants of Restless Legs Syndrome in Pregnancy: A Prospective Study." *Neurology* 80 (February 2013): 738–42. http://www.ncbi.nlm.nih.gov/pubmed/23390174.

Hall, J. G. "When Is Careless Conception a Form of Child Abuse? Lessons from Maternal Phenylketonuria." *The Journal of Pediatrics* 136 (January 2000): 12–3. http://www.ncbi.nlm.nih.gov/pubmed/10636967.

Halsey, Lewis G., and Mike A. Stroud. "100 Years Since Scott Reached the Pole: A Century of Learning About the Physiological Demands of Antarctica." *Physiological Reviews* 92 (April 2102): 521–36. http://www.ncbi.nlm.nih.gov/pubmed/22535890.

Hansen, L., S. M. Sobol, and T. I. Abelson. "Otolaryngologic Manifestations of Pregnancy." *The Journal of Family Practice* 23 (August 1986): 151–5. http://www.ncbi.nlm.nih.gov/pubmed/3525737.

Harden, Cynthia L., and Nitin K. Sethi. "Epileptic Disorders in Pregnancy: An Overview." *Current Opinion in Obstetrics & Gynecology* 20 (December 2008): 557–62. http://www.ncbi.nlm.nih.gov/pubmed/18989131.

Hasan, Reem, Donna D. Baird, Amy H. Herring, Andrew F. Olshan, Michele L. Jonsson Funk, and Katherine E. Hartmann. "Association Between First-Trimester Vaginal Bleeding and Miscarriage." *Obstetrics and Gynecology* 114 (October 2009): 860–7. http://www.pubmedcentral.nih.gov/articlerender .fcgi?artid=2828396&tool=pmcentrez&rendertype=abstract.

Hawfield, Amret, and Barry I. Freedman. "Pre-eclampsia: The Pivotal Role of the Placenta in Its Pathophysiology and Markers for Early Detection." *Therapeutic Advances in Cardiovascular Disease* 3 (February 2009): 65–73. http://www.pubmedcentral.nih.gov/articlerender .fcgi?artid=2752365&tool=pmcentrez&rendertype=abstract.

Hayee, Bu'Hussain, and Ian Forgacs. "Psychological Approach to Managing Irritable Bowel Syndrome." *BMJ* 334 (May 2007): 1105–9. http://www.pubmedcentral.nih.gov/articlerender .fcgi?artid=1877909&tool=pmcentrez&rendertype=abstract.

Hay-Smith, Jean, Siv Morkved, Kate A. Fairbrother, and G. Peter Herbison. "Pelvic Floor Muscle Training for Prevention and Treatment of Urinary and Faecal Incontinence in Antenatal and Postnatal Women." *The Cochrane Database of Systematic Reviews* (January 2008): CD007471. http://www.ncbi.nlm.nih.gov/pubmed/18843750.

Heitkemper, Margaret M., and Lin Chang. "Do Fluctuations in Ovarian Hormones Affect Gastrointestinal Symptoms in Women with Irritable Bowel Syndrome?" *Gender Medicine* 6, (January 2009): 152–67. http://www.pubmedcentral.nih.gov/articlerender .fcgi?artid=3322543&tool=pmcentrez&rendertype=abstract.

Helewa, Michael, Pierre Levesque, Diane Provencher, Robert H. Lea, Vera Rosolowich, and Heather M. Shapiro. "Breast Cancer, Pregnancy, and Breastfeeding." *Journal of Obstetrics and Gynaecology Canada: JOGC* 24 (February 2002): 164–80; quiz 181–4. http://www.ncbi .nlm.nih.gov/pubmed/12196882.

Holbrook, Jaimee, Julia Minocha, and Anne Laumann. "Body Piercing." *American Journal of Clinical Dermatology* 13 (February 2012): 1–17. http://www.ncbi.nlm.nih.gov/pubmed/22175301.

Houston, Laura E., Anthony O. Odibo, and George A. Macones. "The Safety of Obstetrical Ultrasound: A Review." *Prenatal Diagnosis*29 (December 2009): 1204–12. http://www.ncbi.nlm.nih.gov /pubmed/19899071.

Howard, Jo, and Eugene Oteng-Ntim. "The Obstetric Management of Sickle Cell Disease." *Best Practice & Research. Clinical Obstetrics & Gynaecology* 26 (February 2012): 25–36. http://www.ncbi.nlm.nih .gov/pubmed/22113135.

Howell, Emily R. "Pregnancy-Related Symphysis Pubis Dysfunction Management and Postpartum Rehabilitation: Two Case Reports." *The Journal of the Canadian Chiropractic Association* 56 (June 2012): 102–11. http://www.pubmedcentral.nih.gov/articlerender.fcgi ?artid=3364059{\&}tool=pmcentrez{\&}rendertype=abstract.

Hrnjakovic-Cvjetkovic, I., V. Jerant-Patic, D. Cvjetkovic, E. Mrdja, and V. Milosevic. "Congenital Toxoplasmosis." *Medicinski Pregled* 51 (March–April 1998):140–5. http://www.ncbi.nlm.nih.gov/pubmed/9611957.

Iancu, I., M. Kotler, B. Spivak, M. Radwan, and A. Weizman. "Psychiatric Aspects of Hyperemesis Gravidarum." *Psychotherapy and Psychosomatics* 61 (January 1994): 143–9. http://www.ncbi.nlm.nih.gov /pubmed/8066151.

Ilhan, Atilla, Ahmet Gurel, Ferah Armutcu, Suat Kamisli, Mustafa Iraz, Omer Akyol, and Suleyman Ozen. "Ginkgo Biloba Prevents Mobile Phone-Induced Oxidative Stress in Rat Brain." *Clinica Chimica Acta: International Journal of Clinical Chemistry* 340 (February 2004): 153–62. http://www.ncbi.nlm.nih.gov/pubmed/14734207.

Incaudo, Gary A. "Diagnosis and Treatment of Allergic Rhinitis and Sinusitis During Pregnancy and Lactation." *Clinical Reviews in Allergy & Immunology* 27 (October 2004): 159–77. http://www.ncbi.nlm.nih .gov/pubmed/15576899.

Incaudo, Gary A. and Patricia Takach. "The Diagnosis and Treatment of Allergic Rhinitis During Pregnancy and Lactation." *Immunology and Allergy Clinics of North America* 26 (February 2006): 137–54. http:// www.ncbi.nlm.nih.gov/pubmed/16443148.

Jarnfelt-Samsioe, A., G. Samsioe, and G. M. Velinder. "Nausea and Vomiting in Pregnancy: A Contribution to Its Epidemiology." *Gynecologic and*

Obstetric Investigation 16 (January 1983): 221–9. http://www
.ncbi.nlm.nih.gov/pubmed/6629143.

Jewell, D., and G. Young. "Interventions for Nausea and Vomiting in Early
Pregnancy." *The Cochrane Database of Systematic Reviews* (January
2003): CD000145. http://www.ncbi.nlm.nih.gov/pubmed/14583914.

Jin, Fangli, Mingbo Cao, Yangqiu Bai, Yanrui Zhang, Yuxiu Yang, and
Bingyong Zhang. "Therapeutic Effects of Plasma Exchange for the
Treatment of 39 Patients with Acute Fatty Liver of Pregnancy." *Discov-
ery Medicine* 13 (May 2012): 369–73. http://www.ncbi.nlm.nih
.gov/pubmed/22642918.

Kaaja, Risto J., and Ian A. Greer. "Manifestations of Chronic Disease
During Pregnancy." *JAMA* 294 (December 2005): 2751–7. http://www
.ncbi.nlm.nih.gov/pubmed/16333011.

Kafaei Atrian, Mahboobeh, Zohre Sadat, Mahbobeh Rasolzadeh Bid-
goly, Fatemeh Abbaszadeh, and Mohammad Asghari Jafarabadi.
"The Association of Sexual Intercourse During Pregnancy with
Labor Onset." *Iranian Red Crescent Medical Journal* 17 (January 2015): e16465. http://www.pubmedcentral.nih.gov/articlerender
.fcgi?artid=4341500&tool=pmcentrez&rendertype=abstract.

Kalkunte, Satyan, Zhongbin Lai, Wendy E. Norris, Linda A. Pietras, Neetu
Tewari, Roland Boij, Stefan Neubeck, Udo R. Markert, and Suren-
dra Sharma. "Novel Approaches for Mechanistic Understanding and
Predicting Preeclampsia." *Journal of Reproductive Immunology* 83
(December 2009): 134–8. http://www.pubmedcentral.nih.gov
/articlerender .fcgi?artid=2790420&tool=pmcentrez&rendertype
=abstract.

Kalkwarf, Heidi J., and Bonny L. Specker. "Bone Mineral Changes During
Pregnancy and Lactation." *Endocrine* 17 (February 2002): 49–54.
http://www.ncbi.nlm.nih.gov/pubmed/12014704.

Kanakaris, Nikolaos K., Craig S. Roberts, and Peter V. Giannoudis. "Pregnancy-Related Pelvic Girdle Pain: An Update." *BMC Medicine* 9 (January 2011): 15. http://www.pubmedcentral.nih.gov/articlerender
.fcgi?artid=3050758&tool=pmcentrez&rendertype=abstract.

Katz, Vern L., Richard M. Farmer, and Deborah Dotters. "Focus on Primary
Care: From Nevus to Neoplasm: Myths of Melanoma in Pregnancy."
Obstetrical & Gynecological Survey 57 (February 2002): 112–9. http://
www.ncbi.nlm.nih.gov/pubmed/11832787.

Kazmierczak, Maria, Bogumiła Kielbratowska, and Beata Past-
wa-Wojciechowska. "Couvade Syndrome Among Polish
Expectant Fathers." *Medical Science Monitor: International Medical Journal of Experimental and Clinical Research* 19 (January 2013): 132–8. http://www.pubmedcentral.nih.gov/articlerender
.fcgi?artid=3628883&tool=pmcentrez&rendertype=abstract.

Kemmett, D., and M. J. Tidman. "The Influence of the Menstrual Cycle and
Pregnancy on Atopic Dermatitis." *The British Journal of Dermatology*
125 (July 1991): 59–61. http://www.ncbi.nlm.nih.gov/pubmed/1873205.

Khashan, Ali S., Eamonn M. M. Quigley, Roseanne McNamee, Fergus P.
McCarthy, Fergus Shanahan, and Louise C. Kenny. "Increased Risk of
Miscarriage and Ectopic Pregnancy Among Women with Irritable Bowel
Syndrome." *Clinical Gastroenterology and Hepatology: The Official Clin-
ical Practice Journal of the American Gastroenterological Association* 10
(August 2012): 902–9. http://www.ncbi.nlm.nih.gov
/pubmed/22373726.

Kiondo, P., G. Welishe, J. Wandabwa, G. Wamuyu-Maina, G. S.
Bimenya, P. Okong. "Plasma Vitamin C Concentration in Pregnant Women with Pre-eclampsia in Mulago Hospital, Kam-
pala, Uganda." *African Health Sciences* 11 (December 2011):
566–72. http://www.pubmedcentral.nih.gov/articlerender
.fcgi?artid=3362966&tool=pmcentrez&rendertype=abstract.

Kirschbaum, Clemens, Antje Tietze, Nadine Skoluda, and Lucia Det-
tenborn. "Hair as a Retrospective Calendar of Cortisol Production—
Increased Cortisol Incorporation into Hair in the Third Trimester of
Pregnancy." *Psychoneuroendocrinology* 34 (January 2009): 32–7. http://
www.ncbi.nlm.nih.gov/pubmed/18947933.

Kluger, Nicolas. "Body Art and Pregnancy." *European Journal of Obstetrics & Gynecology and Reproductive Biology* 153 (November 2010): 3–7.
http://www.ncbi.nlm.nih.gov/pubmed/20557995.

Kondrackiene, Jūrate, and Limas Kupcinskas. "Liver Diseases Unique to
Pregnancy." *Medicina* 44 (Kaunas, Lithuania, January 2008): 337–45.
http://www.ncbi.nlm.nih.gov/pubmed/18541949.

Koren, Gideon. "Is Air Travel in Pregnancy Safe?" *Canadian Family
Physician: Médecin de famille canadien* 54 (September 2008):

1241–2. http://www.pubmedcentral.nih.gov/articlerender
.fcgi?artid=2553461&tool=pmcentrez&rendertype=abstract.

Kovacs, Christopher S. "Calcium and Bone Metabolism During Pregnancy
and Lactation." *Journal of Mammary Gland Biology and Neoplasia* 10
(April 2005): 105–18. http://www.ncbi.nlm.nih.gov/pubmed/16025218.

Kroumpouzos, G., and L. M. Cohen. "Dermatoses of Pregnancy." *Journal of
the American Academy of Dermatology* 45 (July 2001): 1–19; quiz 19–22.
http://www.ncbi.nlm.nih.gov/pubmed/11423829.

Kroumpouzos, George, and Lisa M. Cohen. "Specific Dermatoses of Pregnancy: An Evidence-Based Systematic Review." *American Journal of
Obstetrics and Gynecology* 188 (April 2003): 1083–92. http://www
.ncbi.nlm.nih.gov/pubmed/12712115.

Kuga, Mutsumi, Minoru Ikeda, Kunio Suzuki, and Shigeo Takeuchi.
"Changes in Gustatory Sense During Pregnancy." *Acta Otolaryngologica
Supplementum* (January 2002): 146–53. http://www.ncbi.nlm
.nih.gov/pubmed/12132613.

Kuhl, C., and J. J. Holst. "Plasma Glucagon and the Insulin:Glucagon Ratio
in Gestational Diabetes." *Diabetes* 25 (January 1976): 16–23. http://
www.ncbi.nlm.nih.gov/pubmed/1245265.

Kvorning, Nina, Catharina Holmberg, Lars Grennert, Anders Åberg, and
Jonas Åkeson. "Acupuncture Relieves Pelvic and Low-Back Pain in Late
Pregnancy." *Acta Obstetricia et Gynecologica Scandinavica* 83 (2004):
246–250. http://www.ncbi.nlm.nih.gov/pubmed/14995919.

Lackner, Jeffrey M., Christina Mesmer, Stephen Morley, Clare Dowzer, and
Simon Hamilton. "Psychological Treatments for Irritable Bowel Syndrome: A Systematic Review and Meta-Analysis." *Journal of Consulting
and Clinical Psychology* 72 (December 2004): 1100–13. http://www
.ncbi.nlm.nih.gov/pubmed/15612856.

Laibl, Vanessa, and Sheffield, Jeanne. "The Management of Respiratory
Infections During Pregnancy." *Immunology and Allergy Clinics of North
America* 26 (February 2006): 155–72. http://www.ncbi.nlm
.nih.gov/pubmed/16443149.

Lao, Michael R., Bryon C. Calhoun, Luis A. Bracero, Ying Wang, Dara J.
Seybold, Mike Broce, and Christos G. Hatjis. "The Ability of the Quadruple Test to Predict Adverse Perinatal Outcomes in a High-Risk Obstetric

Population." *Journal of Medical Screening* 16, no. 2 (June 2009): 55–9. http://www.ncbi.nlm.nih.gov/pubmed/19564516.

Laplante, P. "The Couvade Syndrome: The Biological, Psychological, and Social Impact of Pregnancy on the Expectant Father." *Le Médecin de familie canadien* [Canadian Family Physician] 37 (July 1999): 1633–60. http://www.pubmedcentral.nih.gov/articlerender.fcgi?artid= 2145200&tool=pmcentrez&rendertype=abstract.

Lebel, David E., Ruslan Sergienko, Arnon Wiznitzer, Gad J. Velan, and Eyal Sheiner. "Mode of Delivery and Other Pregnancy Outcomes of Patients with Documented Scoliosis." *The Journal of Maternal-Fetal and Neonatal Medicine* 25, no. 6 (June 2012): 639–41. http://www .ncbi.nlm.nih.gov/pubmed/22070615.

Lee, A. and M. L. Done. "Stimulation of the Wrist Acupuncture Point P6 for Preventing Postoperative Nausea and Vomiting." *The Cochrane Database of Systematic Reviews* (January 2004): http://www.ncbi .nlm.nih.gov/pubmed/15266478.

Lee, R.M. and R.M. Silver. "Recurrent Pregnancy Loss: Summary and Clinical Recommendations." *Seminars in Reproductive Medicine* 18, no. 4 (January 2000): 433–40. http://www.ncbi.nlm.nih.gov /pubmed/11355802.

Leemans, L., "Does 5-methyltetrahydrofolate Offer Any Advantage over Folic Acid?" *Journal de Pharmacie de Belgique* (December 2012): 16–22. http://www.ncbi.nlm.nih.gov/pubmed /23350208.

Lens, M. B. "Effect of Pregnancy on Survival in Women with Cutaneous Malignant Melanoma." *Journal of Clinical Oncology* 22, no. 21 (November 2004): 4369–75. http://www.ncbi.nlm.nih.gov/pubmed/15514378.

Leung, D. T. and S. L. Sacks. "Current Recommendations for the Treatment of Genital Herpes." *Drugs* 60, no. 6 (December 2000): 1329–52. http:// www.ncbi.nlm.nih.gov/pubmed/11152015.

Levy, H. L. and M. Ghavami. "Maternal Phenylketonuria: A Metabolic Teratogen." *Teratology* 53, no. 3 (March 1996): 176–84. http://www .ncbi.nlm.nih.gov/pubmed/8761885.

Li, Jingru, John McCormick, Alan Bocking, and Gregor Reid. "Importance of Vaginal Microbes in Reproductive Health." *Reproductive Sciences* 19, no. 3 (March 2012): 235–42 http://www.ncbi.nlm.nih.gov /pubmed/22383775.

Li, Xiu-Min, and Laverne Brown. "Efficacy and Mechanisms of Action of Traditional Chinese Medicines for Treating Asthma and Allergy." *The Journal of Allergy and Clinical Immunology* (February 2009): 123(2). 297–306; quiz 307. http://www.pubmedcentral.nih.gov/articlerender. fcgi ?artid=2748395&tool=pmcentrez&rendertype=abstract.

Lim, B., E. Manheimer, L. Lao, E. Ziea, J. Wisniewski, J. Liu, and B. Berman. "Acupuncture for Treatment of Irritable Bowel Syndrome." *The Cochrane Database of Systematic Reviews* (January 2006): 4 CD005111. http://www.ncbi.nlm.nih.gov/pubmed/17054239.

Liu, Juntao, Yan Zhao, Yijun Song, Wen Zhang, Xuming Bian, Jianqiu Yang, Dongzhou Liu, Xiaofeng Zeng, and Fengchun Zhang. "Pregnancy in Women with Systemic Lupus Erythematosus: a Retrospective Study of 111 Pregnancies in Chinese Women." *The Journal of Maternal-fetal & Neonatal Medicine: The Official Journal of the European Association of Perinatal Medicine, the Federation of Asia and Oceania Perinatal Societies, the International Society of Perinatal Obstetricians* (March 2012): 261–6. 25(3). http://www.ncbi.nlm.nih.gov/pubmed/21504337.

Longo, L. D. "Maternal Blood Volume and Cardiac Output During Pregnancy: A Hypothesis of Endocrinologic Control." *The American Journal of Physiology* (November 1983): 5 Pt 1, R720—245. http://www .ncbi.nlm.nih.gov/pubmed/6356942.

Louik, Carol, Katherine Ahrens, Stephen Kerr, Junhee Pyo, Christina Chambers, Kenneth L. Jones, Michael Schatz, and Allen A. Mitchell. "Risks and Safety of Pandemic H1N1 Influenza Vaccine in Pregnancy: Exposure Prevalence, Preterm Delivery, and Specific Birth Defects." *Vaccine* (October: 2013): 31(44), 5033–40. http://www.ncbi.nlm.nih .gov/pubmed/24016804.

Loutfy, Mona R., and Sharon L. Walmsley. "Treatment of HIV Infection in Pregnant Women: Antiretroviral Management Options." *Drugs* (January 2004) 64(5) 471–88. http://www.ncbi.nlm.nih.gov/pubmed/14977385.

Lucas, M. J. "Diabetes Complicating Pregnancy." *Obstetrics and Gynecology Clinics of North America* (September 2001): 28(3). 513–36. http:// www.ncbi.nlm.nih.gov/pubmed/11512498.

Lv Lv, Nan, Lan Xiao, and Jun Ma. "Dietary Pattern and Asthma: A Systematic Review and Meta-analysis. *Journal of Asthma and Allergy*

(January 2014): 12:7. 105–21. http://www.pubmedcentral.nih.gov/articlerender .fcgi?artid=4137988&tool=pmcentrez&rendertype=abstract.

Marker-Hermann, Elisabeth, and Rebecca Fischer-Betz. "Rheumatic Diseases and Pregnancy." *Current Opinion in Obstetrics & Gynecology* (December 2010): 22(6). 458–65. http://www.ncbi.nlm.nih.gov /pubmed/20966752.

Muller-Lissner, Stefan A., Michael A. Kamm, Carmelo Scarpignato, and Arnold Wald. "Myths and Misconceptions About Chronic Constipation. *The American Journal of Gastroenterology* (January 2005): 100(1). 232–42. http://www.ncbi.nlm.nih.gov/pubmed/15654804.

MacGregor, E. Anne. "Headache in Pregnancy." *Neurologic Clinics* (August 2012): 30(3). 835–66. http://www.ncbi.nlm.nih.gov /pubmed/22840792.

MacLennan, A. H. "Relaxin—a Review." *The Australian & New Zealand Journal of Obstetrics & Gynaecology* (November 1981): 21(4). 195–202. http://www.ncbi.nlm.nih.gov/pubmed/6280666.

Madhavan Nair, Krishnapillai, Padibidri Bhaskaram, Nagalla Balakrishna, Punjal Ravinder and Boindala Sesikeran. "Response of Hemoglobin, Serum Ferritin, and Serum Transferrin Receptor During Iron Supplementation in Pregnancy: A Prospective Study." *Nutrition (Burbank, Los Angeles County, Calif.)* (October 2004): 20(10). 896–9. http://www .ncbi.nlm.nih.gov/pubmed/15474878.

Mahadevan, Shriraam, R. Bharath, and V. Kumaravel. "Calcium and Bone Disorders in Pregnancy." *Indian Journal of Endocrinology and Metabolism* (May 2012): 16(3). 358–63. http://www.pubmedcentral.nih.gov /articlerender.fcgi?artid=3354840&tool=pmcentrez&rendertype =abstract.

Mandel, L. and K. Tamari. "Sialorrhea and Gastroesophageal Reflux." *Journal of the American Dental Association* (November 1995): 126(11). 1537–41. http://www.ncbi.nlm.nih.gov/pubmed/7499651.

Manheimer, Eric, Ke Cheng, Susan L. Wieland, Li Shih Min, Xueyong Shen, Brian M. Berman, and Lixing Lao. "Acupuncture for Treatment of Irritable Bowel Syndrome." *The Cochrane Database of Systematic Reviews* (January 2012) 16(5). CD005111. http://www.pubmedcentral.nih.gov/articlerender .fcgi?artid=3718572&tool=pmcentrez&rendertype=abstract.

Marques, Mariana, Sandra Bos, Maria Joao Soares, Berta Maia, Ana Telma Pereira, Jose Valente, Ana Allen Gomes, Antonio Macedo, and Maria Helena Azevedo. "Is Insomnia in Late Pregnancy a Risk Factor for Postpartum Depression/Depressive Symptomatology?" *Psychiatry Research* (April 2011):186(2–3). 272–80. http://www.ncbi.nlm.nih .gov /pubmed/20638730.

Maslova, Ekaterina, Sayanti Bhattacharya, Shih-Wen Lin, and Karin B. Michels. "Caffeine Consumption During Pregnancy and Risk of Preterm Birth: A Meta-analysis." *The American Journal of Clinical Nutrition* (November 2010): 92(5). 1120–32. http://www.pubmedcentral.nih.gov/articlerender .fcgi?artid=2954446&tool=pmcentrez&rendertype=abstract.

Massey, E. W. "Carpal Tunnel Syndrome in Pregnancy." *Obstetrical & Gynecological Survey* (March 1978): 33(3). 145–8. http://www.ncbi.nlm .nih.gov/pubmed/343016.

Mastorakos, George, and Ioannis Ilias. "Maternal and Fetal Hypothalamic-Pituitary-Adrenal Axes During Pregnancy and Postpartum." *Annals of the New York Academy of Sciences* (November 2003): 997; 136–49. http://www.ncbi.nlm.nih.gov/pubmed/14644820.

Matalon, Kimberlee Michals, Phyllis B. Acosta, and Colleen Azen. "Role of Nutrition in Pregnancy with Phenylketonuria and Birth Defects." *Pediatrics* (December 2003): 112(6 Pt 2). 1534–6. http://www.ncbi .nlm.nih .gov/pubmed/14654660.

Mazziotti, G. and L. Premawardhana, A. Parkes, H. Adams, P. Smyth, D. Smith, W. Kaluarachi, C. Wijeyaratne, A. Jayasinghe, D. de Silva, J. Lazarus. "Evolution of Thyroid Autoimmunity During Iodine Prophylaxis—the Sri Lankan Experience." *European Journal of Endocrinology* (August 2003): 149(2). 103–110. http://www.eje-online.org/con- tent/149/2/103.abstract.

McCollough, Cynthia H., Beth A. Schueler, Thomas D. Atwell, Natalie N. Braun, Dawn M. Regner, Douglas L. Brown, and Andrew J. LeRoy. "Radiation Exposure and Pregnancy: When Should We Be Concerned?" *Radiographics: A Review Publication of the Radiological Society of North America, Inc.* (July-August 2007): 27(4). 909–17; Discussion 917–8. http://www.ncbi.nlm.nih.gov/pubmed/17620458.

Mezger, N., F. Chappuis, and L. Loutan. "Travelling When Pregnant? Possible, but..." *Revue Médicale Suisse* (May 2005): 1(19). 1263–6. http://www.ncbi.nlm.nih.gov/pubmed/15962623.

Miller, Kevin C., Gary W. Mack, and Kenneth L. Knight. "Gastric Emptying After Pickle-Juice Ingestion in Rested, Euhydrated Humans." *Journal of Athletic Training* (November–December 2010): 45(6). 601–8. http://www.pubmedcentral.nih.gov/articlerender.fcgi?artid=2978012&tool=pmcentrez&rendertype=abstract.

Milman, Nils. "Iron and Pregnancy—a Delicate Balance." *Annals of Hematology* (September 2006): 85(9). 559–65. http://www.ncbi.nlm.nih.gov/pubmed/16691399.

Milman, Nils. "Prepartum Anaemia: Prevention and Treatment." *Annals of Hematology* (December 2008): 87(12). 949–59. http://www.ncbi.nlm.nih.gov/pubmed/18641987.

Milman, N., T. Bergholt, K. E. Byg, L. Eriksen, and N. Graudal. "Iron Status and Iron Balance During Pregnancy. A Critical Reappraisal of Iron Supplementation." *Acta Obstetricia et Gynecologica Scandinavica* (October 1999): 78(9). 749–57. http://www.ncbi.nlm.nih.gov/pubmed/10535335.

Milman, Nils, Thomas Bergholt, Lisbeth Eriksen, Keld-Erik Byg, Niels Graudal, Palle Pedersen, and Jens Hertz. "Iron Prophylaxis During Pregnancy– How Much Iron Is Needed? A Randomized Dose- Response Study of 20-80 mg Ferrous Iron Daily in Pregnant Women." *Acta obstetricia et gynecologica Scandinavica* (March 2005): 84(3). 238–47. http://www.ncbi.nlm.nih.gov/pubmed/15715531.

Milman, Nils, Keld-Erik Byg, Thomas Bergholt, and Lisbeth Eriksen. "Side Effects of Oral Iron Prophylaxis in Pregnancy—Myth or Reality?" *Acta Haematologica* (January 2006): 115(1–2). 53–7. http://www.ncbi.nlm.nih.gov/pubmed/16424650.

Milman, Nils, Keld-Erik Byg, Thomas Bergholt, Lisbeth Eriksen, and Anne-Mette Hvas. "Body Iron and Individual Iron Prophylaxis in Pregnancy—Should the Iron Dose Be Adjusted According to Serum Ferritin?" *Annals of Hematology* (September 2006): 85(9). 567–73. http://www.ncbi.nlm.nih.gov/pubmed/16733739.

Moleski, Stephanie M., and Cuckoo Choudhary. "Special Considerations for Women with IBD." *Gastroenterology Clinics of North America* (June

2011): 40(2). 387–98, viii–ix. http://www.ncbi.nlm.nih.gov
/pubmed/21601786.

Morin, C. M., P. J. Hauri, C. A. Espie, A. J. Spielman, D. J. Buysse, and
R. R. Bootzin. "Nonpharmacologic Treatment of Chronic Insomnia.
An American Academy of Sleep Medicine Review." *Sleep* (December
1999):15; 22(8). 1134–56. http://www.ncbi.nlm.nih.gov
/pubmed/10617176.

Mujezinovic, Faris, and Zarko Alfirevic. "Procedure-Related Complications
of Amniocentesis and Chorionic Villous Sampling." *Obstetrics & Gynecology* (September 2007): 110(3). 687–94. http://www.ncbi.nlm
.nih.gov/pubmed/17766619.

Mustafa, Reem, Sana Ahmed, Anu Gupta, and Rocco C. Venuto. "A Comprehensive Review of Hypertension in Pregnancy." *Journal of Pregnancy*
(January 2012):105918. http://www.pubmedcentral.nih.gov/articleren-
der .fcgi?artid=3366228&tool=pmcentrez&rendertype=abstract.

Naef, R. W., J. R. Allbert, E. L. Ross, B. M. Weber, R. W. Martin, and J. C.
Morrison. "Premature Rupture of Membranes at 34 to 37 Weeks' Gestation: Aggressive Versus Conservative Management." *American Journal of Obstetrics and Gynecology* (January 1998): 178(1 Pt 1). 126–30.
http://www.ncbi.nlm.nih.gov/pubmed/9465815.

Nappi, Rossella E., Francesca Albani, Grazia Sances, Erica Terreno, Eman-
uela Brambilla, and Franco Polatti. "Headaches During Pregnancy."
Current Pain and Headache Reports (August 2011): 15(4). 289–94.
http://www.ncbi.nlm.nih.gov/pubmed/21465113.

Nash, Zachary, Bassem Nathan, and Lawrence Mascarenhas. "Kielland's
Forceps. From Controversy to Consensus?" *Acta Obstetricia et Gynecologica Scandinavica* (January 2015): 94(1). 8–12. http://www.ncbi
.nlm.nih.gov/pubmed/25233861.

Nassar, Anwar H., Dibe Martin, Victor Hugo Gonzalez-Quintero, Orlando
Gomez-Marin, Fawwaz Salman, Alfredo Gutierrez, and Mary J. O'Sul-
livan. "Genetic Amniocentesis Complications: Is the Incidence Over-
rated?" *Gynecologic and Obstetric Investigation* (June 2004): 58(2).
100–4. http://www.ncbi.nlm.nih.gov/pubmed/15178899.

Neely, Anthony L. "Essential Oil Mouthwash (EOMW) May Be Equivalent to Chlorhexidine (CHX) for Long-Term Control of Gingival Inflammation but CHX Appears to Perform Better than EOMW in Plaque

Control." *The Journal of Evidence-Based Dental Practice* (December 2011): 11(4). 171–4. http://www.ncbi.nlm.nih.gov/pubmed/22078823.

Nelson-Piercy, C. "Treatment of Nausea and Vomiting in Pregnancy. When Should It Be Treated and What Can Be Safely Taken?" *Drug Safety* (August 1998): 19(2). 155–64. http://www.ncbi.nlm.nih.gov /pubmed/9704251.

Nisar, Pasha J., and John H. Scholefield. "Managing Haemorrhoids." *BMJ (Clinical Research Ed.)* (October 2003): 11; 327(7419). 847–51. http://www.pubmedcentral.nih.gov/articlerender .fcgi?artid=214027&tool=pmcentrez&rendertype=abstract.

Nitsch-Osuch, Aneta, Agnieszka Wozniak Kosek, and Lidia Bernadeta Brydak. "Vaccination Against Influenza in Pregnant Women—Safety and Effectiveness." *Ginekologia Polska* (January 2013): 84(1). 56–61. http://www.ncbi.nlm.nih.gov/pubmed/23488311.

Obeid, Rima, Wolfgang Holzgreve, and Klaus Pietrzik. "Is 5-methyltetrahydrofolate an Alternative to Folic Acid for the Prevention of Neural Tube Defects?" *Journal of Perinatal Medicine* (September 2013): 41(5). 469–83. http://www.ncbi.nlm.nih.gov/pubmed/23482308.

Obstetrics and Gynecology. "Air Travel During Pregnancy." ACOG Committee Opinion No. 443: (October 2009): 954–5. http://www.ncbi.nlm .nih.gov/pubmed/19888065.

Obstetrics and Gynecology. "Gestational Diabetes." ACOG Practice Bulletin. Number 30, September 2001. http://www.ncbi.nlm.nih.gov /pubmed/11547793.

Okun, Nan, Karen A. Gronau, and Mary E. Hannah. "Antibiotics for Bacterial Vaginosis or Trichomonas Vaginalis in Pregnancy: a Systematic Review." *Obstetrics and Gynecology* (April 2005): 105(4). 857–68. http://www.ncbi.nlm.nih.gov/pubmed/15802417.

Othman, M., J. P. Neilson, and Z. Alfirevic. "Probiotics for Preventing Preterm Labour." *The Cochrane Database of Systematic Reviews* (January 2007): 24(1); CD005941. http://www.ncbi.nlm.nih.gov /pubmed/17253567.

Ozguner, Fehmi, Ahmet Altinbas, Mehmet Ozaydin, Abdullah Dogan, Huseyin Vural, A. Nesimi Kisioglu, Gokhan Cesur, and Nurhan Gumral Yildirim. "Mobile Phone-induced Myocardial Oxidative Stress: Protection by a Novel Antioxidant Agent Caffeic Acid Phenethyl Ester."

Toxicology and Industrial Health (October 2005): 21(9). 223–30.
http://www.ncbi.nlm.nih.gov/pubmed/16342473.

Padmanabhan, Rengasamy. "Etiology, Pathogenesis and Prevention of
Neural Tube Defects." *Congenital Anomalies* (June 2006): 46(2). 55–67.
http://www.ncbi.nlm.nih.gov/pubmed/16732763.

Padua, Luca, Antonella Di Pasquale, Costanza Pazzaglia, Giovanna A.
Liotta, Alessia Librante, and Mauro Mondelli. "Systematic Review of
Pregnancy-Related Carpal Tunnel Syndrome." *Muscle & Nerve* (November 2010): 42(5). 697–702. http://www.ncbi.nlm.nih.gov
/pubmed/20976778.

Parkes, Ilana L., Joseph G. Schenker, and Yoel Shufaro. "Thyroid Disorders
During Pregnancy." *Gynecological Endocrinology: the Official Journal
of the International Society of Gynecological Endocrinology* (December
2012): 28(12). 993–8. http://www.ncbi.nlm.nih.gov/pubmed/22686167.

Patrick, L. "Comparative Absorption of Calcium Sources and Calcium
Citrate Malate for the Prevention of Osteoporosis." *Alternative Medicine Review: a Journal of Clinical Therapeutic* (April 1999): 4(2). 74–85.
http://www.ncbi.nlm.nih.gov/pubmed/10231607.

Patterson, William L., and Georgel, Philippe T. "Breaking the Cycle: the
Role of Omega-3 Polyunsaturated Fatty Acids in Inflammation-Driven
Cancers." *Biochemistry and Cell Biology = Biochimie et Biologie Cellulaire* (October 2014): 92(5). 321–8. http://www.ncbi.nlm.nih.gov
/pubmed/25098909.

Pereira, Adriana, and Bruce P. Krieger. "Pulmonary Complications of Pregnancy." *Clinics in Chest Medicine* (June 2004): 25(2). 299–310. http://
www.ncbi.nlm.nih.gov/pubmed/15099890.

Perkins, J., R. L. Hammer, and P. V. Loubert. "Identification and Management of Pregnancy-Related Low Back Pain." *Journal of Nurse-Midwifery* (September–October 1998): 43(5). 331—40. http://www.ncbi
.nlm.nih.gov/pubmed/9803711.

Pfab, F., J. Huss-Marp, A. Gatti, J. Fuqin, G. I. Athanasiadis, D. Irnich, U.
Raap, W. Schober, H. Behrendt, J. Ring, and U. Darsow. "Influence of
Acupuncture on Type I Hypersensitivity Itch and the Wheal and Flare
Response in Adults with Atopic Eczema - a Blinded, Randomized, Placebo-controlled, Crossover Trial." *Allergy* (July 2010): 65(7). 903–10.
http://www.ncbi.nlm.nih.gov/pubmed/20002660.

Pfab, F., M. T. Kirchner, J. Huss-Marp, T. Schuster, P. C. Schalock, J. Fuqin, G. I. Athanasiadis, H. Behrendt, J. Ring, U. Darsow, and V. Napadow. "Acupuncture Compared with Oral Antihistamine for Type I Hypersensitivity Itch and Skin Response in Adults with Atopic Dermatitis: A Patient- and Examiner-Blinded, Randomized, Placebo-Controlled, Crossover Trial." *Allergy* (April 2012): 67(4). 566–73. http://www.pubmedcentral.nih.gov/articlerender.fcgi?artid=3303983&tool=pmcentrez&rendertype=abstract.

Plagemann, A., T. Harder, R. Kohlhoff, W. Rohde, and G. Dorner. "Overweight and Obesity in Infants of Mothers with Long-Term Insulin-Dependent Diabetes or Gestational Diabetes." *International Journal of Obesity and Related Metabolic Disorders: Journal of the International Association for the Study of Obesity* (June 1997): 451–6. http://www.ncbi.nlm.nih.gov/pubmed/9192228.

Powe, Camille E., Cheryl D. Knott, and Nancy Conklin-Brittain. "Infant Sex Predicts Breast Milk Energy Content." *American Journal of Human Biology: The Official Journal of the Human Biology Council* (2010): 50–4. http://www.ncbi.nlm.nih.gov/pubmed/19533619.

Puliyath, G., and S. Singh. "Leptospirosis in Pregnancy." *European Journal of Clinical Microbiology and Infectious Diseases* (May 2012): 2491–6. http://www.ncbi.nlm.nih.gov/pubmed/22549729.

Quigley, E. M., and B. Flourie. "Probiotics and Irritable Bowel Syndrome: a Rationale for Their Use and an Assessment of the Evidence to Date." *Neurogastroenterology and Motility* (March 2007): 166–172. http://www.ncbi.nlm.nih.gov/pubmed/17300285.

Rădulescu, Micaela, Emil Coriolan Ulmeanu, Mihaela Nedelea, and Andrei Oncescu. "Prenatal Ultrasound Diagnosis of Neural Tube Defects." Prenatal Ultrasound. Pictorial Essay. (2012). http://www.ncbi.nlm.nih.gov/pubmed/22675716.

Rasmussen, Kathleen M., Ann L. Yaktine, Institute of Medicine (US), and National Research Council (US) Committee to Reexamine IOM Pregnancy Weight Guidelines. *Weight Gain During Pregnancy*. Washington (DC): National Academies Press, 2009. http://www.ncbi.nlm.nih.gov/books/NBK32813.

Reid, Gregor, and Alan Bocking. "The Potential for Probiotics to Prevent Bacterial Vaginosis and Preterm Labor." *American Journal of Obstetrics*

and Gynecology (October 2003): 1202–8. http://www.ncbi.nlm.nih.gov
/pubmed/14586379.

Reynolds, Tim. "The Triple Test as a Screening Technique for Down Syndrome: Reliability and Relevance." *International Journal of Women's
Health* (January 2010): 83–8. http://www.pubmedcentral.nih.gov
/articlerender .fcgi?artid=2971727&tool=pmcentrez&rendertype
=abstract.

Richter, J. E. "Review Article: the Management of Heartburn in Pregnancy." *Alimentary Pharmacology and Therapeutics* (November 2005):
749–57. http://www.ncbi.nlm.nih.gov/pubmed/16225482.

Riely, Caroline A., and Yannik Bacq. "Intrahepatic Cholestasis of Pregnancy." *Clinics in Liver Disease* (February 2004): 167–76. http://www
.ncbi.nlm.nih.gov/pubmed/15062199.

Ross, Mary Elizabeth, Peter E. Waldron, William J. Cashore, Pedro A. de
Alarcon, Eric Werner, and Robert D. Christensen. *Neonatal Hematology*. New York: Cambridge University Press, 2012.

Rothenberg, Karen H. *Women and Prenatal Testing: Facing the Challenges
of Genetic Technology*. Ohio State University Press, 1994.

Rouse, B., R. Matalon, R. Kock, C. Azen, H. Levy, W. Hanley, F. Trefz, and
F de la Cruz. "Maternal Phenylketonuria Syndrome: Congenital Heart
Defects, Microcephaly, and Developmental Outcomes. *The Journal of
Pediatrics* (January 2000): 57–61. http://www.ncbi.nlm.nih.gov
/pubmed/10636975.

Sabino, Jennifer, and Jonathan N. Grauer. "Pregnancy and Low Back Pain."
Current Reviews in Musculoskeletal Medicine (June 2008): 137–41.
http://www.pubmedcentral.nih.gov/articlerender.
fcgi?artid=2684210&tool=pmcentrez&rendertype=abstract.

Sahota, Pradeep K., Sanjay S. Jain, and Rajiv Dhand. "Sleep Disorders
in Pregnancy." *Current Opinion in Pulmonary Medicine* (November
2003): 477–83. http://www.ncbi.nlm.nih.gov/pubmed/14534398.

Sanz, Yolanda. "Gut Microbiota and Probiotics in Maternal and Infant
Health." *The American Journal of Clinical Nutrition* (December 2011):
2000S-2005S. http://www.ncbi.nlm.nih.gov/pubmed/21543533.

Sastre, Juan, Ana Lloret, Consuelo Borras, Javier Pereda, David Gar-
cia-Sala, Marie-Therese Droy-Lefaix, Federico V. Pallardo, and Jose
Vina. "Ginkgo Biloba Extract EGb 761 Protects Against Mitochondiral

Aging in the Brain and Liver." *Cellulary and Molecular Biology* (Noisy-le-Grand, France). (September 2002): 685–92. http://www.ncbi.nlm .nih.gov/pubmed/12396080.

Sastre, J., F. V. Pallardo, J. Garcia de la Asuncion, and J. Vina. "Mito-chondira, Oxidative Stress and Aging." (March 2000): 189–98. http:// www.ncbi.nlm.nih.gov/pubmed/10730818.

Sepulveda, W., E. Corral, C. Ayala, C. Be, J. Gutierrez, and P. Vasquez. "Chromosomal Abnormalities in Fetuses with Open Neural Tube Defects: Prenatal Identification with Ultrasound." *The Official Journal of the International Society of Ultrasound in Obstetrics and Gynecology* (April 2004): 352–6. http://www.ncbi.nlm.nih.gov/pubmed/15065184.

Shapiro, Eugene D. "Lyme Disease." *The New England Journal of Medicine* (August 2014): 371. http://www.pubmedcentral.nih.gov/articlerender .fcgi?artid=4492124&tool=pmcentrez& rendertype=abstract.

Sheiner, Eyal, and Jacques S. Abramowicz. "A Symposium on Obstetri-cal Ultrasound: Is All This Safe for the Fetus?" Clinical Obstetrics and Gynecology (March 2012): 188–98. http://www.ncbi.nlm.nih.gov /pubmed/22343238.

Sheiner, Eyal, Moshe Mazor, Amalia Levy, Arnon Wiznitzer, and Asher Bashiri. "Pregnancy Outcome of Asthmatic Patients: a Population-Based Study." *The Journal of Maternal-Fetal and Neonatal Medicine* (October 2005): 37–40. http://www.ncbi.nlm.nih.gov/pubmed/16318973.

Sheiner, E., I. Shoham-Vardi, M. Hallak, R. Hershkowitz, M. Katz, and M. Mazor. "Placenta Previa: Obstetric Risk Factors and Pregnancy Out-come." *The Journal of Maternal-Fetal Medicine* (December 2001): 414–9. http://www.ncbi.nlm.nih.gov/pubmed/11798453.

Sheiner, Eyal, Illana Vardi-Shoham, Michael J. Hussey, Xavier Pombar, Howard T. Strassner, Jody Freeman, and Jacques S Abramowicz. "First-Trimester Sonography: Is the Fetus Exposed to High Levels of Acoustic Energy?" *Journal of Clinical Ultrasound: JCU* (June 2007): 245–9. http://www.ncbi.nlm.nih.gov/pubmed/17410588.

Shen, Yi-Hao, and Richard Nahas. "Complementary and Alternative Medi-cine for Treatment of Irritable Bowel Syndrome." Canadian Family Phy-sician (February 2009): 143–8. http://www .pubmedcentral.nih.gov /articlerender.fcgi?artid=2642499&tool = pmcentrez&rendertype=abstract.

Shimanovich, Iakov, Eva B. Brocker, and Detlef Zillikens. "Pemphigoid Gestationis: New Insights into the Pathogenesis Lead to Novel Diagnostic Tools." *BJOG: An International Journal of Obstetrics and Gynaecology* (September 2002): 970–6. http://www.ncbi.nlm.nih.gov/pubmed/12269691.

Shornick, J. K., J. L. Bangert, R. G. Freeman, and J. N. Gilliam. "Herpes Gestationis: Clinical and Histologic Features of Twenty-Eight Cases." *Journal of the American Academy of Dermatology* (February 1983): 214–24. http://www.ncbi.nlm.nih.gov/pubmed/6338065.

Sipiora, M. L., M. A. Murtaugh, M. B. Gregoire, and V. B. Duffy. "Bitter Taste Perception and Severe Vomiting in Pregnancy." Physiology and Behavior (May 2000): 259–67. http://www.ncbi.nlm.nih.gov/pubmed/10869591.

Smith, A. David, Young-In Kim, and Helga Refsum. "Is Folic Acid Good for Everyone?" *The American Journal of Clinical Nutrition* (March 2008): 517–33. http://www.ncbi.nlm.nih.gov/pubmed/18326588.

Smith, Graeme N., Ian Gemmill, and Kieran M. Moore. "Management of Tick Bites and Lyme Disease During Pregnancy." *Journal of Obstetrics and Gynaecology Canada* (November 2012): 1087–91. http://www.ncbi.nlm.nih.gov/pubmed/23231847.

Smyth, Andrew, Guilherme H. M. Oliveira, Brian D. Lahr, Kent R. Bailey, Suzanne M. Norby, and Vesna D. Garovic. "A Systematic Review and Meta-Analysis of Pregnancy Outcomes in Patients with Systemic Lupus Erythematosus and Lupus Nephritis." *Clinical Journal of the American Society of Nephrology: CJASN* (November 2010): 2060–8. http://www.pubmedcentral.nih.gov/articlerender.fcgi?artid=3001786&tool=pmcentrez&rendertype=abstract.

Snell, B. J. "Assessment and Management of Bleeding in the First Trimester of Pregnancy." *Journal of Midwifery and Women's Health* (January 2009): 483–91. http://www.ncbi.nlm.nih.gov/pubmed/19879521.

Soheilykhah, Sedigheh, Mahdieh Mojibian, Maryam Rashidi, Soodabeh Rahimi-Saghand, and Fatemeh Jafari. "Maternal Vitamin D Status in Gestational Diabetes Mellitus." *Nutrition in Clinical Practice: Official Publication of the American Society for Parenteral and Enteral Nutrition* (October 2010): 524–7. http://ncp.sagepub.com/content/25/5/524.abstract. http://www.ncbi.nlm.nih.gov/pubmed/20962313.

Sokolovic, Dusan, Boris Djindjic, Jelenka Nikolic, Gordana Bjelakovic, Dusica Pavlovic, Gordana Kocic, Dejan Krstic, Tatjana Cvetkovic, and Voja Pavlovic. "Melatonin Reducses Oxidative Stress Induced by Chronic Exposure of Microwave Radiation from Mobile Phones in Rat Brain." *Journal of Radiation Research* (November 2008): 579–86. http://www.ncbi.nlm.nih.gov/pubmed/18827438.

Sosa, Claudio G., Fernando Althabe, Jose M. Belizan, and Eduardo Bergel. "Bed Rest in Singleton Pregnancies for Preventing Preterm Birth." *The Cochrane Database of Systematic Reviews* (January 2015): CD003581. http://www.ncbi.nlm.nih.gov/pubmed/25821121.

Sripramote, Manit, and Nol Lekhyanada. "A Randomized Comparison of Ginger and Vitamin B6 in the Treatment of Nausea and Vomiting of Pregnancy." *Journal of the Medical Association of Thailand* (2003): 846–53. http://www.ncbi.nlm.nih.gov/pubmed/14649969.

Staples, Judith, Anne-Louise Ponsonby, and Lynette Lim. "Low Maternal Exposure to Ultraviolet Radiation in Pregnancy, Month of Birth, and Risk of Multiple Sclerosis in Offspring: Longitudinal Analysis." *BMJ* (Clinical research ed.) (2010): c1640. http://www.pubmedcentral.nih.gov/articlerender.fcgi?artid=2862149&tool=pmcentrez&rendertype=abstract.

Stearns, S. *Maternal Effects as Adaptations*. Oxford University Press, 1999.

Stockton, Susan, Karen Breshears, and David M. Baker. "The Impact of a Food Elimination Diet on Collegiate Athletes' 300-Meter Run Time and Concentration." *Global Advances in Health and Medicine: Improving Healthcare Outcomes Worldwide* (November 2014): 25–40. http://www.pubmedcentral.nih.gov/articlerender.fcgi?artid=4268641&tool=pmcentrez&rendertype=abstract.

Stone, J. L., and C. J. Lockwood. "Amniocentesis and Chorionic Villus Sampling." *Current Opinion in Obstetrics and Gynecology* (1993): 211–7. http://www.ncbi.nlm.nih.gov/pubmed/8490091.

Straface, Gianluca, Alessia Selmin, Vincenzo Zanardo, Marco De Santis, Alfredo Ercoli, and Giovanni Scambia. "Herpes Simplex Virus Infection in Pregnancy." *Infectious Diseases in Obstetrics and Gynecology* (January 2012): 385697. http://www.pubmedcentral.nih.gov/articlerender.fcgi?artid=3332182&tool=pmcentrez&rendertype=abstract.

Stuart, Mari, and Linda Bergstom. "Pregnancy and Multiple Sclerosis." *Journal of Midwifery and Women's Health* (January 2011): 41–7. http://www.ncbi.nlm.nih.gov/pubmed/21323849.

Studd, J., and N. Panay. "Chronic Fatigue Syndrome." *Lancet* (November 1996): 1384. http://www.ncbi.nlm.nih.gov/pubmed/8918295.

Stuge, Britt, Gunvor Hilde, and Nina Vollestad. "Physical Therapy for Pregnancy-Related Low Back and Pelvic Pain: A Systematic Review." *Acta Obstetricia et Gynecologica Scandinavica* (November 2003): 983–90. http://www.ncbi.nlm.nih.gov/pubmed/14616270.

Suzuki, Shunji, Miwa Igarashi, Eriko Yamashita, and Misao Satomi. "Ptyalism Gravidarum." *North American Journal of Medical Sciences* (November 2009): 303–4. http://www.pubmedcentral.nih.gov/articlerender.fcgi?artid=3364630&tool=pmcentrez&rendertype=abstract.

Taubel, M., M. Sulyok, V. Vishwanath, E. Bloom, M. Turunen, K. Jarvi, E. Kauhanen, R. Krska, A. Hyvarinen, L. Larsson, and A. Nevalainen. "Co-occurrence of Toxic Bacterial and Fungal Secondary Metabolites in Moisture-Damaged Indoor Environments." *Indoor Air* (October 2011): 368–75. http://www.ncbi.nlm.nih.gov/pubmed/21585551.

Tai, Shusheng, Jiulin Wang, Feng Sun, Stevenson Xutian, Tianshan Wang, and Malcolm King. "Effect of Needle Puncture and Electro-Acupuncture on Mucociliary Clearance in Anesthetized Quails." *BMC Complementary and Alternative Medicine* (January 2006): 4. http://www.pubmedcentral.nih.gov/articlerender.fcgi?artid=1397865&tool=pmcentrez&rendertype=abstract.

Tan, Peng C., and Siti Z. Omar. "Contemporary Approaches to Hyperemesis During Pregnancy." *Current Opinion in Obstetrics and Gynecology* (April 2011): 87–93. http://www.ncbi.nlm.nih.gov/pubmed/21297474.

Taylor, Nicholas. "Transient False-Positive Urine Human Chorionic Gonadotropin in Septic Shock." *The American Journal of Emergency Medicine* (June 2015): 864.e1-2. http://www.ncbi.nlm.nih.gov/pubmed/25616588.

Teissier, Raphael, Emmanuel Nowak, Murielle Assoun, Karine Mention, Cano Aline, Alain Fouilhoux, Fraccois Feillet, Helene Ogier, Emmanuel Oger, and Loice de Parscau. "Maternal Phenylketonuria: Low Phenylalaninemia Might Increase the Risk of Intra Uterine Growth Retardation."

Journal of Inherited Metabolic Disease (November 2012): 993–9. http://www.ncbi.nlm.nih.gov/pubmed/22669364.

Ter Haar, Gail. "Ultrasonic Imaging: Safety Conditions." *Interface Focus* (August 2011): 686–97. http://www.pubmedcentral.nih.gov/articlerender.fcgi?artid=3262273&tool=pmcentrez&rendertype =abstract.

Thomas, R. G. R., and W. A. Liston. "Clinical Associations of Striae Gravidarum." *Journal of Obstetrics and Gynaecology: The Journal of the Institute of Obstetrics and Gynaecology* (April 2004): 270–1. http://www.ncbi.nlm.nih.gov/pubmed/15203623.

Thomas, Sanjeev V. "Managing Epilepsy in Pregnancy." *Neurology India* 59–65. http://www.ncbi.nlm.nih.gov/pubmed/21339661.

Thrasher, J. D., and S. Crawley. "The Biocontaminants and Complexity of Damp Indoor Spaces: More than What Meets the Eye." *Toxicology and Industrial Health* (September 2009): 583–615. http://www.ncbi.nlm .nih.gov/pubmed/19793773.

Triche, Elizabeth W., Laura M. Grosso, Kathleen Belanger, Amy S. Darefsky, Neal L. Benowitz, and Michael B. Bracken. "Chocolate Consumption in Pregnancy and Reduced Likelihood of Preeclampsia." *Epidemiology* (May 2008): 459–64. http://www.pubmedcentral.nih.gov/articlerender .fcgi?artid=2782959&tool=pmcentrez&rendertype=abstract.

Tunzi, Marc, and Gary R. Gray. "Common Conditions During Pregnancy." *American Family Physician* (January 2007): 211–8. http://www .ncbi.nlm.nih.gov/pubmed/17263216.

Vambergue, A., A. S. Valat, P. Dufour, M. Vazaubiel, P. Fontaine, and F. Puech. "Pathophysiology of Gestational Diabetes." *Journal de Gynecologie, Obstetrique, et Biologie de la Reproduction* (October 2002): 4S3–4S10. http://www.ncbi.nlm.nih.gov/pubmed/12451352.

Van Dinter, M. C. "Pytalism in Pregnant Women." *Journal of Obstetric, Gynecologic, and Neonatal Nursing: JOGNN/NAACOG* (May–June 1991): 206–9. http://www.ncbi.nlm.nih.gov/pubmed/2056357.

Vleeming, Andry, Hanne B. Albert, Hans Christian Ostgaard, Bengt Sturesson, and Britt Stuge. "European Guidelines for the Diagnosis and Treatment of Pelvic Girdle Pain." *European Spine Journal* (February

2008): 794–819. http://www.pubmedcentral.nih.gov/articlerender
.fcgi?artid=2518998&tool=pmcentrez&rendertype=abstract.

Vogell, Alison, Rupsa C. Boelig, Joanna Skora, and Jason K. Baxter. "Bilateral Bell Palsy as a Presenting Sign of Preeclampsia." *Obstetrics and Gynecology* (August 2014): 459–61. http://www.ncbi.nlm.nih.gov
/pubmed/25004308.

Vojdani, Aristo, Frank Hebroni, Yaniv Raphael, Jonathan Erde, and Bernard Raxlen. "Novel Diagnosis of Lyme Disease: Potential for CAM Intervention." *Evidence-Based Complementary and Alternative Medicine*: *eCAM* (September 2009): 283–95. http://www.pubmedcentral.nih.gov/articlerender
.fcgi?artid=2722197&tool=pmcentrez&rendertype=abstract.

Wang, Chi Chiu, Lu Li, Ling Yin Tang, and Ping Chung Leung. "Safety Evaluation of Commonly Used Chinese Herbal Medicines During Pregnancy in Mice." *Human Reproduction* (Oxford, England). (August 2012): 2448–56.

Warren, Lucie, Jaynie Rance, and Billie Hunter. "Feasibility and Acceptability of a Midwife-Led Intervention Programme Called 'Eat Well Keep Active' to Encourage a Healthy Lifestyle in Pregnancy." *BMC Pregnancy and Childbirth* (January 2012): 27. http://www.pubmedcentral.nih.gov/articlerender
.fcgi?artid=3354634&tool=pmcentrez&rendertype=abstract.

Wei, Juan, Xitong Zhang, Yang Bi, Ruidong Miao, Zhong Zhang, and Hailan Su. "Anti-Inflammatory Effects of Cumin Essential Oil by Blocking JNK, ERK, and NF- Signaling Pathways in LPS-Stimulated RAW 264.7 Cells." *Evidence-Based Complementary and Alternative Medicine* (January 2015): 474509. http://www.pubmedcentral.nih.gov/articlerender .fcgi?artid=4575746&tool=pmcentrez&rendertype=abstract.

West, L., J. Warren, and T. Cutts. "Diagnosis and Management of Irritable Bowel Syndrome, Constipation, and Diarrhea in Pregnancy." *Gastroenterology Clinics of North America*. (December 1992): 793–802.

Widnes, Sofia Frost, Jan Schjott, and Anne Gerd Granas. "Risk Perception and Medicines Information Needs in Pregnant Women with Epilepsy—a Qualitative Study." *Seizure: the Journal of the British Epilepsy Association* (October 2012): 597–602. http://www.ncbi.nlm.nih.gov
/pubmed/22762859.

Wilson, Danielle L., Maree Barnes, Lenore Ellett, Michael Permezel, Martin Jackson, and Simon F Crowe. "Decreased Sleep Efficiency, Increased Wake After Sleep Onset and Increased Cortical Arousals in Late Pregnancy." *The Australian and New Zealand Journal of Obstetrics and Gynaecology* (February 2011): 38–46. http://www.ncbi.nlm.nih.gov/pubmed/21299507.

Winer, N. "Different Methods for the Induction of Labour in Postterm Pregnancy." *Journal de Gynecologie, Obstetrique, et Biologie de la Reproduction* (December 2011): 796–811. http://www.ncbi.nlm.nih.gov/pubmed/22056188.

Wjst, Matthias. "Is Vitamin D Supplementation Responsible for the Allergy Pandemic?" *Current Opinion in Allergy and Clinical Immunology* (June 2012): 257–62. http://www.ncbi.nlm.nih.gov/pubmed/22517291.

Wong, R. C., and C. N. Ellis. "Physiologic Skin Changes in Pregnancy." *Journal of the American Academy of Dermatology* (June 1984): 929–40. http://www.ncbi.nlm.nih.gov/pubmed/6376552.

Young, G. L., and D. Jewell. "Interventions for Preventing and Treating Pelvic and Back Pain in Pregnancy." *The Cochrane Database of Systematic Reviews* (January 2002): CD001139. http://www.ncbi.nlm.nih.gov/pubmed/11869592.

———. "Creams for Preventing Stretch Marks in Pregnancy." *The Cochrane Database of Systematic Reviews* (September 1996): CD000066. http://www.ncbi.nlm.nih.gov/pubmed/10796111.

———. "Interventions fo Varicosities and Leg Oedema in Pregnancy." *The Cochrane Database of Systematic Reviews* (January 2000): CD001066. http://www.ncbi.nlm.nih.gov/pubmed/10796237.

———. "Topical Treatment for Vaginal Candidiasis (Thrush) in Pregnancy." *The Cochrane Database of Systematic Reviews* (January 2001): CD000225. http://www.ncbi.nlm.nih.gov/pubmed/11687074.

———. "Interventions for Leg Cramps in Pregnancy." *The Cochrane Database of Systematic Reviews* (January 2002): CD000121. http://www.ncbi.nlm.nih.gov/pubmed/11869565.

Zhang, C., S. Liu, C. G. Solomon, and F. B. Hu. "Dietary Fiber Intake, Dietary Glycemic Load, and the Risk for Gestational Diabetes Mellitus." *Diabetes Care* (September 2006): 2223–30. http://www.ncbi.nlm.nih.gov/pubmed/17003297.

Zhang, C., M. B. Schulze, C. G. Solomon, and F. B. Hu. "A Prospective Study of Dietary Patterns, Meat Intake, and the Risk of Gestational Diabetes Mellitus." *Diabetologia* (November 2006): 2604–13. http://www.ncbi.nlm.nih.gov/pubmed/16957814.

Zhang, Jun, Mario Merialdi, Lawrence D. Platt, and Michael S. Kramer. "Defining Normal and Abnormal Fetal Growth: Promises and Challenges." *American Journal of Obstetrics and Gynecology* (June 2010): 522–8. http://www.pubmedcentral.nih.gov/articlerender.fcgi?artid=2878887&tool=pmcentrez&rendertype=abstract.

Zioni, Tammy, Dan Buskila, Barak Aricha-Tamir, Arnon Wiznitzer, and Eyal Sheiner. "Pregnancy Outcome in Patients with Fibromyalgia Syndrome." *The Journal of Maternal-Fetal and Neonatal Medicine* (November 2011): 1325–8. http://www.ncbi.nlm.nih.gov/pubmed/21284491.

Index

About the Author

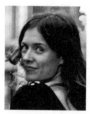 CAYLIE SEE, MS, LAC, (FABORM), is a board-licensed acupuncturist and herbalist with over two decades of experience guiding women into successful pregnancies. She has often heard the phrase: "I knew it would be challenging being pregnant, but nobody told me [fill in the blank]." She wrote this book to fill in those blanks for readers. Her passion lies in seeing women through the full-spectrum of their pregnancy experience—especially the challenging parts. She believes that underneath these rocky places lies the very information that women need to feel fully supported and understood.

In addition to her extensive clinical experience in women's health, See has held teaching positions at esteemed academic institutions such as the California Institute of Integral Studies and Acupuncture and Integrative Medicine College, Berkeley. She is also widely published in peer-reviewed research including the *Journal of Clinical Oncology* and the *Journal of Complementary and Alternative Medicine*. She is currently the executive director of Integrative Fertility and was the founding vice president of the American Board of Oriental Reproductive Medicine.

See is also a new mother, an experience that has greatly illuminated these pages.